ENDOSCOPIC ULTRASOUND - FROM USUAL TO SPECIAL

Edited by **Charing Chong**

Endoscopic Ultrasound - From Usual to Special
http://dx.doi.org/10.5772/62925
Edited by Charing Chong

Contributors

Amir Houshang Mohammad Alizadeh, Khaled Bamakhrama, Abed Al-Lehibi, Ilya Sivokozov, Olga Lovacheva, Irina Shabalina, Galina Evgushenko, Larisa Lepekha, Yuri Berezovsky, Larisa Chernousova, Elena Larionova, Tatyana Statsuk, Natalya Makaryants, Lidia Ciobanu, Radu Ion Badea, Lucio Giovanni Battista Rossini, Juliana Marques Drigo, Gisele De Fatima Cordeiro Leite

Published by InTech

Janeza Trdine 9, 51000 Rijeka, Croatia

Publishing Process Manager Dajana Pemac

Technical Editor SPi Global

Cover InTech Design team

First published February, 2017
Printed in Croatia

Additional hard copies can be obtained from orders@intechopen.com

Endoscopic Ultrasound - From Usual to Special, Edited by Charing Chong
p. cm.
Print ISBN 978-953-51-2939-4
Online ISBN 978-953-51-2940-0

For EU product safety concerns:
IN TECH d.o.o., Prolaz Marije Krucifikse Kozulić 3, 51000 Rijeka, Croatia,
info@intechopen.com or visit our website at intechopen.com.

Meet the editor

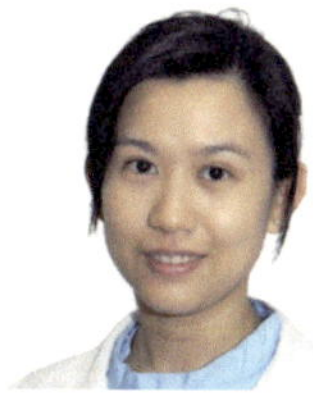

Dr. Charing Chong, MBChB, MSc, FRCSEd (Gen. Surg.), is currently a clinical assistant professor at the Department of Surgery of the Chinese University of Hong Kong. She is the principal or coinvestigator for a variety of clinical and preclinical studies examining new approaches for the treatment of liver and pancreatic cancer and endoscopic ultrasound. Dr. Chong serves as an editor and reviewer in various journals. She also serves as subcommittee of standardization of teaching material in the Asian EUS Group and she is also a member of various profession societies including the Hong Kong Society of Hepatobiliary and Pancreatic Surgery, Hong Kong Society of Minimal Access Surgery, Hong Kong Society of Robotic Surgery and Hong Kong Society of Digestive Endoscopy.

Contents

Preface

Endoscopic ultrasound (EUS) has been introduced in clinical practice since 1980 (DiMagno EP 1980)[1]. During the past few decades, the application of this instrument has been extended tremendously. EUS is able to provide direct visualization beyond the walls of gastrointestinal tract, and fine-needle aspiration is extremely useful for the diagnosis of benign and malignant disease of adjacent structures, for example the mediastinum, pancreas and pelvic organs, that may be difficult to reach otherwise. In the recent years, reports on the basic principles and applications of EUS in upper gastrointestinal and pancreaticobiliary diseases have been extensively published. This book provides an overview of endoscopic ultrasound, from usual to special applications.

This book provides the readers with an update on some usual applications of EUS such as pancreatic cysts and subepithelial lesions. On the other hand, this book also provides insight into several interesting special clinical applications, such as endobronchial ultrasound in mediastinal lymphadenopathy, endoluminal ultrasonography of the rectum as well as the endoscopic ultrasound and intestinal endometriosis. This book will be valued by surgeons, gastrointestinal and respiratory physicians as well as gynaecologists who strive to know more on the application of EUS.

Charing Chong, MBChB, MSc, FRCSEd(Gen)
Assistant Professor
Division of Hepatobiliary and Pancreatic Surgery
Department of Surgery
Prince of Wales Hospital
The Chinese University of Hong Kong

[1] DiMagno EP, Buxton JL, Regan PT, et al. Ultrasonic endoscope. Lancet 1980;1:629-31. (DiMagno EP, 1980)

Section 1

Common Applications

Chapter 1

The Role of EUS in Pancreatic Cysts

Amir Houshang Mohammad Alizadeh

Additional information is available at the end of the chapter

http://dx.doi.org/10.5772/65126

Abstract

Pancreatic cystic lesions (PCLs) comprise various pathologically different groups of lesions that usually share many common clinical features. Cystic lesions and fluid collections of the pancreas often present a diagnostic and therapeutic challenge. Pancreatic cystic lesions are being diagnosed with increasing frequency owing to the widespread use of cross-sectional imaging. The differential diagnosis for cystic lesions of the pancreas is broad, and the role of endoscopic ultrasonography (EUS) is becoming more clearly defined. EUS has become an important tool in the diagnosis and risk stratification of pancreatic cysts. The ability of EUS to provide detailed imaging, tissue, and cyst fluid for analysis makes it a seemingly powerful diagnostic tool for PCLs. It can accurately visualize the cyst morphology, assess vascular pattern by contrast harmonic scan, and perform fine-needle aspiration (FNA) for evaluation of cytology and molecular markers. Furthermore, several studies have shown the therapeutic applications of endoscopic ultrasound in management of PCLs, including EUS-guided ablation of cystic pancreatic tumors by injection of alcohol, aiding in pancreatic pseudocyst drainage.

Keywords: pancreatic cysts, EUS, IPMN, mucinous cytadenoma, serous cystadenoma

1. Introduction

Pancreatic cystic lesions (PCLs) are being diagnosed with increasing frequency, including a wide spectrum from benign to malignant and invasive lesions. The most commonly observed PCL types include intraductal papillary mucinous neoplasms (IPMN), mucinous cystic neoplasms (MCN), serous cystic neoplasms (SCN), and pseudocysts (PC) [1, 2]. Differentiation of neoplastic mucinous from non-mucinous cysts that are managed quite differently is important. If non-mucinous pancreatic lesions such as inflammatory pseudocysts and neoplastic lesions are accurately characterized, most does not require resection or long-term follow-up. Mucinous neoplasms have a known pre-malignant potential and, therefore, are either resected or monitored in a surveillance program [3, 4].

Preoperative diagnosis of PCLs must be reliable as the current standard treatment, major or total pancreatectomy, dramatically affects quality of life. Additionally, early diagnosis of malignancy is essential to an improved prognosis. Despite being the most common modality to identify cystic pancreatic lesions, cross-sectional imaging plays a variable role in characterizing these lesions. Endoscopic ultrasonography (EUS) has become an important tool in the diagnosis and risk stratification of pancreatic cysts [5–7].

EUS was first introduced by Dr. Eugene DiMagno in the 1980s by combining a high frequency ultrasound transducer to an endoscope. In 1991, convex linear-array echoendoscope was introduced by Pentax. These linear scopes scan parallel to the longitudinal axis of the scope and enable fine-needle aspiration (FNA) and different therapeutic applications. EUS provides real-time high-resolution images of cystic pancreatic lesions with morphological details [6, 8]. The combination of fine-needle aspiration (FNA) cytology with the other recently available diagnostic markers has further increased its diagnostic accuracy. The current diagnostic evaluation of PCL often includes EUS-guided fine-needle aspiration (EUS-FNA) for cyst fluid analysis. In addition to the role of EUS in the differential diagnosis of pancreatic cystic lesions, EUS-FNA is also important in management of cystic tumors of the pancreas [9, 10].

2. Diagnostic role of EUS

The critical issue being faced in routine clinical practice is accurate preoperative characterization of cystic lesions. Histology remains the gold standard but requires resection. Since that is impractical for most low risk lesions, imaging provides indirect evidence of morphology. Pancreatic cysts can be diagnosed and assessed by using computer tomography (CT) and magnetic resonance (MR), but these imaging modalities have been inconsistent in differentiating them [3, 11]. CT scan, MRI, and MRCP are generally considered safe and reliable in providing follow-up data on cyst and pancreatic duct size but are less sensitive in detecting intra-mural nodules, which are better evaluated by EUS-FNA [6, 12]. The accuracy of MRI and CT to make a specific diagnosis is suboptimal, with reports of 39–50 and 40–44%, respectively. Efforts to differentiate pancreatic cystic lesions from imaging tests have met with mixed success, with up to 40% of neoplastic cysts misdiagnosed as pseudocyst [3, 7]. EUS, particularly as a means of EUS-guided cyst aspiration, has become an important tool in the diagnosis and risk stratification of pancreatic cysts. The diagnostic accuracy of EUS for identification of malignant or pre-malignant pancreatic cysts reaches 95%, although this method has significant limitations for the differential diagnosis of benign and malignant cysts with overall accuracy rates of 40–93% [7, 11].

The goal in assessing pancreatic cysts by EUS is to avoid characterizing a mucinous cyst as a benign serous cyst and erroneously opting for simple observation instead of potentially curable surgical resection. Endoscopic ultrasound is increasingly used for the differential diagnosis of pancreatic cystic lesions either alone or in combination with fine-needle aspiration. EUS allows close and high-resolution imaging of cystic pancreatic lesion morphology. The appearances of the cyst wall, the presence of septate or solid components, the number of cysts, and concomitant lymphadenopathy have been used to distinguish between benign and malignant cystic lesions [6, 13]. EUS-FNA has the added advantage of allowing aspiration of the cyst contents and sampling of the cyst wall or septa, as well as mural nodules. Cyst fluid aspiration can be more studied to analyze cytology, tumor markers, enzymes, as well as DNA analysis of DNA quality/content or mutational analysis [9, 14].

2.1. EUS morphology

Some PCLs have a very typical morphology and may thus be easily diagnosed by imaging. Diagnosis based on the findings of EUS requires attention to the number and size of cysts, shapes of whole cysts, state of the cyst wall, internal state of the cysts, communication between the pancreatic duct and the cyst, and existence of any background lesions (**Table 1**). It is generally believed that a differential diagnosis is practicable partly by collating these findings with the above features of the various pancreatic cystic lesions [15, 16].

Cyst type	Location	Morphology/EUS findings	Fluid color and viscosity	Cytology	CEA[1]	Amylase
Mucinous cystadenoma	Body/tail more than head	Macrocystic, occasionally septated; peripheral calcifications, soli components and regional adenopathy when malignant	Colorless, thick fluid	Extracellular mucin. Mucinous epithelial cells may be seen in a background of ovarian stroma	Moderate to very high	Variable
IPMN[2]	Main duct or side branch; head more than body and tail	Dilated main pancreatic duct or side branches; may appear as a septated cyst; may have a solid component	Colorless, thick fluid	Extracellular mucin. Mucinous epithelial cells may be seen with papillary projections and variable atypia	Moderate to very high	Elevated
Serous cystadenoma	Body/tail more than head	Microcystic with a honeycomb appearance; rarely has a macrocystic component; central calcification	Colorless, often contain blood	Typically acellular. Small glycogen staining cuboidal cells in the background may be seen	Undetectable to low	Low
Pseudocyst	Anywhere	Anechoic, thick-walled, rare septa tions, regional inflammatory nodes may be seen	Yellow to brown thin fluid	Macrophages with no mucin. Mixed inflam matory infiltrate may be seen	Low to at least increase	Elevated

[1]Carcinoembryonic antigen.
[2]Intraductal papillary mucinous neoplasm.

Table 1. Characteristics of cyst fluid in the main types of cystic pancreatic lesions [2, 6].

Several EUS findings have been evaluated to diagnose pancreatic cystic lesions. Studies have shown that small cyst size does not exclude malignancy. Some features do appear to be more predictive in diagnosing specific types of cystic lesions. The existence of multiple small compartments (<3 mm) within a cystic lesion (also called a microcystic lesion) is indicative of a serous cystic neoplasm, with an accuracy of 92–96%, and this feature is not seen in mucinous cystadenomas. A cystic lesion without septations or solid components and seen within a pancreas having parenchymal features suggestive of a pseudocyst with sensitivity and specificity of 94 and 85%, respectively. However, EUS morphology alone does not appear to be very reliable to establish a specific diagnosis or to differentiate between benign and malignant diseases (**Figures 1** and **2**) [2, 6, 7].

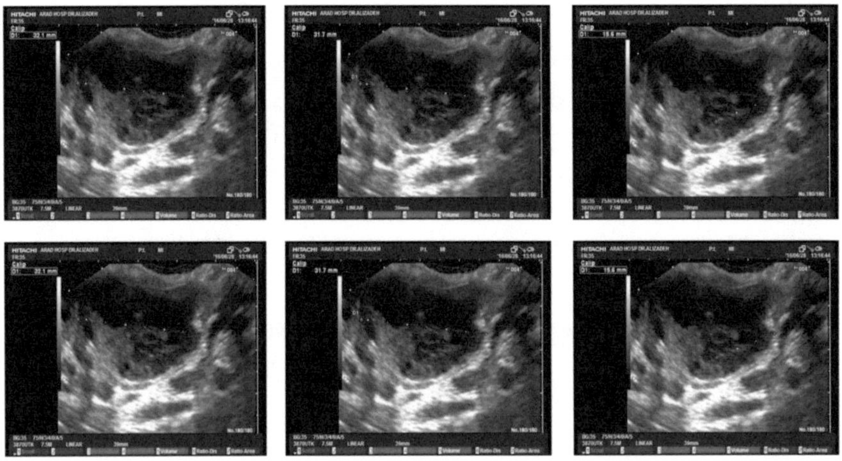

Figure 1. Main-duct intraductal papillary mucinous neoplasm (MD-IPMN): thick wall with mural nodules—by Prof. Alizadeh.

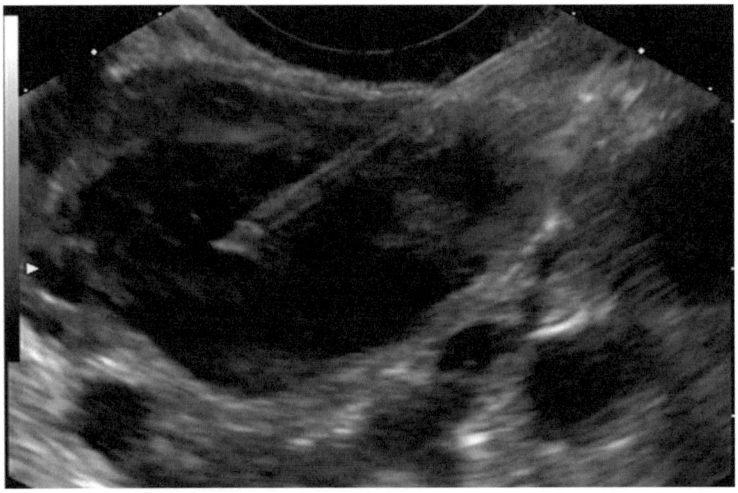

Figure 2. Cyst fluid evaluation-EUS/FNA—by Prof. Alizadeh.

2.2. Cyst fluid evaluation

EUS-FNA allows aspiration of the cyst contents and plays an important role in differential diagnosis of doubtful cases of pancreatic cysts. Cyst fluid analysis is useful in differential diagnosis between mucinous and non-mucinous pancreatic cystic tumors. Cystic fluid aspirate is acellular or with minimal cellularity in up to 72% of aspirated cysts. Cyst fluid can be studied after aspiration to analyze cytology, viscosity, extracellular mucin, tumor markers (CEA, CA 19-9, CA 153, Ca 72-4, etc.), enzymes (amylase, lipase), and DNA analysis. Analysis of cystic fluid aspirate can be used to differentiate mucinous from non-mucinous cysts with a sensitivity, specificity, and accuracy of 12.5–27, 90–100, and 55%, respectively [7, 17].

2.2.1. *EUS-FNA with cyst fluid cytology*

Due to the shortcomings of EUS alone, the use of EUS-FNA has been extensively evaluated for fluid analysis and cytology of pancreatic cystic lesions. EUS-FNA cytology provides excellent specificity (more than 90%) for the diagnosis of cystic pancreatic lesions. However, the sensitivity of EUS-FNA remains widely variable with most studies reporting sensitivity under 50% [6, 7].

EUS-FNA can provide material for a cytologic diagnosis in up to 80% of cases of pancreatic cystic lesions. Viscosity is usually lower in pseudocysts and serous cystadenomas when compared with mucinous cystadenoma and mucinous cystadenocarcinoma. Furthermore, the presence of extracellular mucin in aspirated cyst fluid is moderately predictive of a mucinous neoplasm. Findings suggestive of a pseudocyst include macrophages, histiocytes, and neutrophils. The presence of mucin indicates a mucinous neoplasm and is seen in 35% or more of cases. FNA from a minority of serous cystadenoma may reveal the presence of glycogen-rich cuboidal cells (**Table 1**) [2, 11, 18].

2.2.2. *Cystic fluid analysis and tumor markers*

Because of the limited sensitivity of cytology, cyst fluid may be analyzed for levels of amylase, lipase, and tumor markers, such as carcinoembryonic antigen (CEA) and carbohydrate antigen (CA) 19-9. Early studies in the 1980s suggested the role of CEA and CA 19-9 in the differentiation of pancreatic cystic lesions [9, 18].

Cyst fluid contains glycoproteins, such as CEA, CA 19-9, CA 125, CA 15-3, and CA 72-4, which are secreted from the epithelial lining. CEA is currently considered the most reliable for the diagnosis of mucinous cystic pancreatic lesions. This marker is typically elevated in mucinous lesions but is lower in pseudocysts and non-mucinous tumors [6, 7]. CA 19-9 also has wide overlapping of results with pseudocysts and serous cystadenomas. Furthermore, other markers such as amylase and lipase may be important in the evaluation of cystic pancreatic lesions. Amylase is useful in the differentiation of pseudocysts from cystic neoplasm and usually elevated not only in inflammatory cysts like pseudocysts but also in mucinous neoplasm due to communication with the pancreatic duct (**Table 2**) [6, 9, 13].

Cyst	Viscosity	Amylase	CA 72-4	CEA	CA 15-3	CA 19-9
Pseudocyst	Low	High	Low	Low	Low	Low
Serous cystadenoma	Low	Variable	Low	Low	Low	Low
Mucinous cystadenoma	Often high	Variable	Low	High	High	High
Mucinous cystadenocarcinoma	High	Variable	High	High	High	High

Table 2. Cyst fluid analysis for differentiation of pancreatic cystic lesions [19].

2.2.3. Cystic fluid analysis and genetic markers

Another differential diagnosis of pancreatic cystic lesions is DNA and mutational analysis in the cystic fluid aspirated by EUS-FNA. Molecular analysis of pancreatic cyst aspirated fluid may be helpful in predicting malignancy. The detection of loss of heterozygosity (LOH) by using microsatellite markers closely linked to key tumor suppressor genes can serve as a surrogate marker for gene inactivation and mutation [11, 18].

Molecular markers are greatly sought as a more reliable alternative diagnostic marker for many malignancies, due to the revolution in translational science. Specific genetic markers are increasingly identified and used to measure the risk of malignancy in pancreatic cystic lesions. It is believed that IPMNs should follow a transformation process similar to the adenoma-carcinoma sequence in colon cancer, where hyperplastic lesions progress to dysplastic and carcinoma cells. Recently, the oncogene GNAS was detected in IPMN tissue. Some reports have indicated that GNAS mutations are prevalent especially in the intestinal and invasive form of IPMN. Furthermore, mutations in K-*ras*, *p*16, and *p*53 have been reported in associated with progression of cystic pancreatic lesion from non-dysplastic to dysplastic cysts [6, 7, 18].

3. Therapeutic role of EUS

Management of incidentally detected pancreatic cysts with malignant potential is a common clinical challenge. Surgical resection is the treatment of choice for most suspicious cystic lesions of the pancreas [12, 19]. Surgical resection of pancreatic cyst is associated with a perioperative morbidity rate of 20–40% and a mortality rate of 2%. EUS can be used to mark the optimal puncture site or to perform EUS-guided cyst puncture and drainage. Moreover, EUS-guided anti-tumor therapy may be applied to cystic pancreatic tumors, and early results of EUS-guided alcohol injection into pancreatic cystic tumors were recently reported [2, 10, 19].

3.1. Endoscopic drainage

A pancreatic pseudocyst is the most common cystic lesion of the pancreas. Pseudocysts should be drained when symptomatic, progressively enlarging, or infected. Pseudocysts have been drained through stenting of the pancreatic duct (transpapillary drainage) or stenting of a drainage tract created between the pseudocyst and the gastroduodenal lumen (transmural drainage). Drainage can be achieved through endoscopic, radiologic, or surgical techniques. Endoscopic drainage of pancreatic pseudocysts is less invasive than surgery [14, 20].

Endoscopic methods for pancreatic pseudocyst drainage are associated with low mortality and acceptable success rates. EUS-guided drainage is associated with a low rate of complications. Prior to the availability of EUS, transmural endoscopic cyst drainage was reliant on a combination of radiologic imaging to ensure a distance of less than 10 mm between gastrointestinal lumen and cyst. Endoscopic drainage may be performed as so-called single-step endo-ultrasonography (EUS)-guided and two-(multi)-step EUS-guided drainage techniques [14, 17]. EUS has the theoretical advantage of reducing the risks of bleeding, perforation, and, potentially, infection. Furthermore, this technique can provide important information in aiding pancreatic pseudocyst drainage. It allows accurate measurement of the distance between the gut lumen and the cystic cavity of the pseudocyst. EUS is helpful in identifying debris within a pseudocyst, which may not be drainable and which may increase the risk of infection [21, 22].

3.2. EUS-guided pancreatic cyst ablation

EUS-guided pancreatic cyst ablation is practically an alternative treatment in selected patients who are not candidates for or who refuse surgery. Based on the accumulated experiences of endoscopic ultrasonography-guided fine-needle aspiration (EUS-FNA), EUS-guided pancreatic tissue ablation with ethanol or other ablative agents was performed safely, with few procedure-related complications [12, 23]. Complications of cyst ablation were reported as rare and mild. The most common acute complication was abdominal pain after cyst ablation (7.9%) and acute pancreatitis developed in 2%. Although a novel technique such as radiofrequency ablation was recently reported, it is still unclear whether or not cyst ablation is justified. Safety, efficacy, and cost-effectiveness of EUS-guided pancreatic cyst ablation should be further validated [7, 24].

To date, ethanol (80–99%) and paclitaxel have been investigated as ablative agents in pancreatic cysts. A commonly used ablative agent is ethanol owing to its cost-effectiveness, ready availability, and rapid ablative effect. The low viscosity of ethanol permits repeated filling and emptying of the cyst [7, 23].

Ablation of the epithelial lining of a pancreatic cystic neoplasm has been proposed as a way to reduce or eliminate malignant or metastatic potential in benign and malignant lesions, respectively. Ethanol lavage of MCN and IPMN cystic lesions by using EUS guidance appears to be safe, but its efficacy has not yet been determined. The mechanisms involved in destruction of cyst epithelium include cell membrane lysis, rapid protein precipitation, and vascular occlusion. Treatment response is further supported by adding a chemotherapeutic agent (most commonly paclitaxel), which acts as an inhibitor of the disassembly process of microtubules during cell division and subsequently inducing apoptosis [18, 25].

4. Conclusion

Pancreatic cystic lesions (PCLs) comprise a diverse group of histopathologic bodies possessing varying degrees of malignancy. PCLs range from benign abnormalities needing minimal follow-up to pre-malignant or malignant lesions requiring careful monitoring or resection. The diagnosis and management of pancreatic cystic lesions are a common problem. EUS and EUS-guided fine-needle aspiration (FNA) can play an important role in the differential diagnosis of pancreatic cystic lesions and decision about referral for possible surgery by evaluating cytology and tumor markers. There is some emerging evidence that EUS-guided pancreatic cyst ablation by injection of alcohol can help to treatment of the cystic pancreatic tumors. Furthermore, EUS can provide important information in aiding pancreatic pseudocyst drainage.

Author details

Amir Houshang Mohammad Alizadeh*

Address all correspondence to: ahmaliver@yahoo.com

Endoscopy Department, Research Center for Gastroenterology and Liver Diseases, Taleghani Hospital, Shahid Beheshti University of Medical Sciences, Evin, Tehran, Iran

References

[1] Barresi L, Tarantino I, Granata A, Curcio G, Traina M. Pancreatic cystic lesions: How endoscopic ultrasound morphology and endoscopic ultrasound fine-needle aspiration help unlock the diagnostic puzzle. World Journal of Gastrointestinal Endoscopy. 2012;4(6):247-59.

[2] Jacobson BC, Baron TH, Adler DG, Davila RE, Egan J, Hirota WK, et al. ASGE guideline: The role of endoscopy in the diagnosis and the management of cystic lesions and inflammatory fluid collections of the pancreas. Gastrointestinal Endoscopy. 2005;61(3): 363-70.

[3] Kwon RS, Scheiman JM. EUS and pancreatic cyst fluid analysis: Is the juice worth the aqueeze? Journal of Gastrointestinal Oncology. 2011;2(4):199.

[4] Thiruvengadam N, Park WG. Systematic review of pancreatic cyst fluid biomarkers: The path forward. Clinical and Translational Gastroenterology. 2015;6(6):e88.

[5] Wang Q-X, Xiao J, Orange M, Zhang H, Zhu Y-Q. EUS-guided FNA for diagnosis of pancreatic cystic lesions: A meta-analysis. Cellular Physiology and Biochemistry. 2015;36(3):1197-209.

[6] Al-Haddad M, El Hajj II, Eloubeidi MA. Endoscopic ultrasound for the evaluation of cystic lesions of the pancreas. Journal of the Pancreas. 2010;11(4):299-309.

[7] Kelvin YMC, Park J-S, Seo D-W. Role of endosonography in the management of incidental pancreatic cystic lesions. Gastrointestinal Intervention. 2014;3(1):40-5.

[8] Iqbal S, Friedel D, Gupta M, Ogden L, Stavropoulos SN. Endoscopic-ultrasound-guided fine-needle aspiration and the role of the cytopathologist in solid pancreatic lesion diagnosis. Pathology Research International. 2012;2012.

[9] Rockacya M, Khalida A. Update on pancreatic cyst fluid analysis. Annals of Gastroenterology. 2012;26:1-6.

[10] Bhutani MS. Role of endoscopic ultrasonography in the diagnosis and treatment of cystic tumors of the pancreas. Journal of the Pancreas. 2004;5(4):266-72.

[11] Snow P. Pancreatic cyst fluid analysis – A review. Journal of Gastrointestinal and Liver Diseases. 2011;20(2):175-80.

[12] Oh HC, Seo DW. Endoscopic ultrasonography-guided pancreatic cyst ablation (with video). Journal of Hepato-Biliary-Pancreatic Sciences. 2015;22(1):16-9.

[13] Sand J, Nordback I. The differentiation between pancreatic neoplastic cysts and pancreatic pseudocyst. Scandinavian Journal of Surgery. 2005;94(2):161-4.

[14] Breslin N, Wallace MB. Diagnosis and fine-needle aspiration of pancreatic pseudocysts: The role of endoscopic ultrasound. Gastrointestinal Endoscopy Clinics of North America. 2002;12(4):781-90.

[15] Okabe Y, Kaji R, Ishida Y, Tsuruta O, Sata M. The management of the pancreatic cystic neoplasm: The role of the EUS in Japan. Digestive Endoscopy. 2011;23(s1):39-42.

[16] Jenssen C, Kahl S. Management of incidental pancreatic cystic lesions. Viszeralmedizin. 2015;31(1):14-24.

[17] Jabłońska B. Pancreatic cysts: Etiology, diagnosis and management. Central European Journal of Medicine. 2014;9(1):92-107.

[18] Khalid A, Brugge W. ACG practice guidelines for the diagnosis and management of neoplastic pancreatic cysts. The American Journal of Gastroenterology. 2007;102(10): 2339-49.

[19] Van Dam J. EUS in cystic lesions of the pancreas. Gastrointestinal Endoscopy. 2002;56(4):S91-S3.

[20] Buscail L, Faure P, Bournet B, Selves J, Escourrou J. Interventional endoscopic ultrasound in pancreatic diseases. Pancreatology. 2006;6(1-2):7-16.

[21] Fazel A, Draganov P. Interventional endoscopic ultrasound in pancreatic disease. Current Gastroenterology Reports. 2004;6(2):104-10.

[22] Raj M, Chen RY. Interventional applications of endoscopic ultrasound. Journal of Gastroenterology and Hepatology. 2006;21(2):348-57.

[23] Cho M-K, Choi J-H, Seo D-W. Endoscopic ultrasound-guided ablation therapy for pancreatic cysts. Endoscopic Ultrasound. 2015;4(4):293.

[24] Nakai Y, Isayama H, Itoi T, Yamamoto N, Kogure H, Sasaki T, et al. Role of endoscopic ultrasonography in pancreatic cystic neoplasms: Where do we stand and where will we go? Digestive Endoscopy. 2014;26(2):135-43.

[25] Zhang W-Y, Li Z-S, Jin Z-D. Endoscopic ultrasound-guided ethanol ablation therapy for tumors. World Journal of Gastroenterology. 2013;19(22):3397-403.

Chapter 2

Role of Endoscopic Ultrasound in Subepithelial Lesions (SELs)

Abed Al-Lehibi and Khaled Bamakhrama

Additional information is available at the end of the chapter

http://dx.doi.org/10.5772/67102

Abstract

A subepithelial lesion (SET) is defined as a lesion, bulge or impression visible within the lumen of the gastrointestinal tract that is covered by normally appearing mucosa and usually found incidentally during routine endoscopy. Such a lesion could be either an intramural mass or an impression caused by extramural structures. The old terminology has recently been replaced by the term "subepithelial lesion" because intramural lesions may arise and can be located in any layer of the GI wall underneath the epithelium. The most common SELs are gastrointestinal stromal tumors (GISTs), leiomyomas, lipomas, granular cell tumors (GCTs), pancreatic rests and carcinoid tumors. The prognosis varies from benign to potentially malignant. While the majority of the lesions are considered benign, some tumors such as GISTs and carcinoids have a strong propensity for malignant transformation. Endoscopic ultrasonography (EUS) is the most accurate diagnostic method for distinguishing between extraluminal compressions and intramural lesions and plays a critical role in the detection and management of SELs. This is because EUS can reveal the precise sonographic nature of the lesion even though sometimes there are complex cases, which are difficult to diagnose by EUS alone. Performing routine biopsies and obtaining tissue samples for diagnosis can be difficult because SELs are located beneath the normal epithelial layer. Mostly, EUS allows the practitioner to extract an optimal tissue sample since it allows fine-needle aspiration (FNA) and fine-needle biopsy (FNB) both of which provide good results. With immunocytochemical staining, all these techniques increase the accuracy of the diagnosis. Evaluation of subepithelial lesions by means of EUS imaging will provide further characterization of the lesion to help guide us in appropriate differential diagnosis and further management. In this chapter, we provide a systematic EUS-guided approach to the diagnosis, management and later surveillance for SELs, as well as presenting updated diagnostic techniques that may help physicians to appropriately manage these subepithelial lesions.

Keywords: endoscopy, endoscopic ultrasound (EUS), subepithelial lesion (SET), fine-needle aspiration (FNA), fine-needle biopsy (FNB), multidetector computed tomography (MDCT)

1. Introduction

The prevalence of subepithelial lesions (SELs) detected on routine endoscopy is unknown; however, these are frequently encountered with 0.36% of EGD procedures. During the last 10 years, the detection rate has increased, with advances in endoscopic technology with the more widespread use of EUS and close attention paid during routine endoscopy exams and reported with 1%, with an incidence of 1 in 300 patients [1]. The malignant lesions are reported with 13% accuracy [2]. Men and women are equally affected. Most of the patients are more than 50-year old. Usually US, CT and MRI are not sensitive enough to detect and characterize the majority of SELs since they can be smaller than 1 cm in size. SELs have a wide and diverse spectrum of etiologies (normal structures; benign lesions and malignant tumor), clinical course, radiological, and understanding the endoscopic, EUS and underlying pathologic features of SELs is essential for their detection, differential diagnosis, staging and management. They are most commonly found in the stomach, esophagus and duodenum. The lower GI, rectum, and cecum are the commonest sites. Lipomas can be seen any part of the colon. They mostly occur in the rectum and cecum, but familiar lesions such as lipomas may be seen in any part of the colon. In SELs, the order was as follows: Gastrointestinal stromal tumor (GIST), leiomyoma, hemangioma, external compression, pancreatic rest and granular cell tumor (**Table 1**). Most benign SELs can be diagnosed according to their endoscopic appearance, but findings on routine biopsy are not usually that helpful. Benign SELs tumors have a lower detection rate due to the fact that they are often small and most patients are asymptomatic. A minority of cases present with abdominal pain, vomiting, anemia, dysphagia, or gastrointestinal (GI) bleeding and obstruction, most of which are likely to result from complications and depending on the site and size of the lesion. [3] Among SETs, the malignant potential of GISTs is related to size; however, malignancy can be detected in smaller lesions [4]. However, SETs can have malignant potential, and it is therefore critical to be able to exclude malignant or premalignant lesions [5], the prognoses varying from benign to very aggressive with malignant potential.

Common benign lesions	
1	Lipomas
2	Ectopic pancreas
3	Schwannomas
4	Duplication cysts
Common malignant lesions	
1	GIST
2	Lymphoma
3	Metastasis

Table 1. Differential diagnosis of SELs.

Therefore, proper diagnostic and therapeutic plans are needed for GI SETs. For this purpose, endoscopic ultrasonography (EUS) is the most accurate diagnostic method [6]. The lesion can be evaluated based on its size, layer of origin and echotexture, echogenic homogeneity, and the presence of echogenic and anechoic foci. Border, extension to adjacent layers, irregular margins and invasion into adjacent organs or structures can all be used to help identify intramural lesions or direct further management (surgical resection, endoscopic submucosal resection/dissection) or studies (special stains and immunohistochemical evaluation of tissue samples) [7, 8]. There are some typical findings for some GI SETs such as lipoma, duplication cysts, and ectopic pancreas [7, 9]. However, most hypoechoic SELs make it difficult to come to a final diagnosis using EUS images alone. Biopsy is necessary for the definite diagnosis of GI SETs. Despite obtaining appropriate biopsy specimens, using an endoscopic biopsy procedure is often difficult and inconclusive [10]. To overcome the limitations of conventional endoscopic biopsy methods, using the bite-on-bite biopsy technique [11], EUS-guided cytology or biopsy methods, such as EUS-guided fine-needle aspiration (EUS-FNA), EUS-guided fine-needle biopsy (EUS-FNB) technique, have now been introduced to obtain sufficient tissue. EUS-tissue sampling is a safe procedure for the diagnosis of GI SETs and is used for cytological studies. Immunohistochemical staining (IHS) methods are used, resulting in good diagnostic yields. Recently, EUS-FNB has been introduced and reportedly provides good results for the diagnosis of GI SETs [8]. Although biopsy, including FNA and FNB or excision, is required for a definitive diagnosis. Management is generally based upon the confidence of diagnosis and whether the lesion causes symptoms. With advanced endoscopy technology and the more common use of EUS, the diagnosis and management of SETs has been changed.

2. Endoscopic ultrasound

Radial EUS and mini-probe EUS can reveal the precise nature and provide accurate diagnosis of GI SETs. SETs such as lipoma, duplication cysts, and ectopic pancreas exhibit some typical findings. Forward-viewing linear EUS has been introduced and has been shown to provide good image quality and shorter observation times in SETs than oblique-viewing linear EUS [12, 42]. EUS is the gold standard for evaluation of SELs with high precision. EUS is able to differentiate external compression from intramural lesion and to determine the layer of origin [13, 14]. The echogenicity of lesions is different. We can thus differentiate GISTs, leiomyomas, and schwannomas. The echogenicity of a leiomyoma is equal to the echogenicity of proper muscle, while a GIST shows slightly higher echogenicity than that of the proper muscle, and a schwannoma shows extremely low echogenicity [2]. In addition, EUS is better at providing a more accurate indication of the size of lesion than other modalities. EUS can evaluate for regional lymphadenopathy. Tissue biopsy can be obtained. Finally, EUS helps to determine appropriate management of the case. Some noninvasive imaging methods, such as transabdominal ultrasonography (US), computed tomography (CT), and magnetic resonance imaging (MRI), have been used, but they are often insufficient. With these methods, the transition zone (the area where the tumor arises from normal gut wall layers) needs to be examined carefully to determine the layer of origin. The reported accuracy of EUS in predicting the pathologic diagnosis of subepithelial lesions showed a wide range, from 45.5 to 82.9% [14–19]. The sensitivity and specificity of EUS malignant finding is 64 and 80%, respectively [6]. However, EUS findings are not sufficient to accurately predict malignancy [10]. If tissue was obtained from EUS-guided fine-needle aspiration (EUS-FNA), the diagnostic accuracy increased markedly, ranging from 63 to 98% [1, 26–28]. EUS-FNA for SETs using a forward-viewing linear EUS has provided good results: full histologic assessment rate of 93.4%, sensitivity of 92.8%, specificity of 100% [20, 42]. Tumor size and location are important factors for good sampling in EUS-FNA for GI SETs. The diagnostic rate for tumors ≥4 cm was 100%, but for tumors of 2–4 and <2 cm, the diagnostic rates were only 86% and 71%, respectively [21, 22]. Using cytology alone, differentially diagnosing GISTs from other mesenchymal tumors is not easy. Findings of mitosis in EUS-FNA specimens are known to be associated with malignant GISTs [29, 30], Ki-67 staining is helpful in evaluating the aggressiveness of GISTs [7, 23, 24]. Many studies have reported the use of various EUS-FNA needles to improve diagnostic accuracy. Tissue sampling and diagnostic rates for SETs were similar when comparing the use of 22 and 25 G EUS-FNA needles (sampling rate, sensitivity, positive predictive value, negative predictive value: 100, 55, 100, and 0% for 22 G needles; 100, 64, 100, and 0% for 25 G needles) [25]. Furthermore, 25 G needles were superior to 22 G needles for diagnosing mobile small lesions. A histologic yield of 95% using this needle was similar to the 90% achieved in EUS-FNB using 19 G Pro-Core (Cook Endoscopy, Wilson-Salem, NC, USA) needles [26]. EUS-FNA with an on-site cytopathologist (rapid on-site cytopathological examination) resulted in a 10–29% increase in the adequacy rates of EUS-FNA specimens and a 10–15% increase in the diagnostic rate [27, 28]. Recently, EUS-FNB using reverse bevel cheese slicer technology has been introduced [29]. A study compared 22 G EUS-FNA and 22 G EUS-FNB in EUS-guided GI SET sampling. The EUS-FNB group required a significantly lower number of needle passes than the EUS-FNA group. The EUS-FNB group had higher yields of optimal macroscopic (30% vs. 92%,) and histological (20% vs. 75%,) core samples with three needle passes, which resulted in a high diagnostic rate (20% vs. 75%) [8]. The EUS helps in deciding whether a lesion should be removed or followed in situ [30]. Lesions confined to the mucosal or submucosal layers can be safely removed endoscopically. Surgical resection, if needed, is generally recommended for lesions located in muscularis propria, although these lesions need to be removed by experienced clinicians. There is minimal risk when using advances in endoscopic techniques such as endoscopic submucosal dissection (ESD) [5, 31, 32]. Follow-up EUS is often used in SETs smaller than 2 cm. For small GI SETs, follow-up after a 1-year interval is recommended. If the size of the mass is unchanged during two serial EUS follow-ups, extended follow-up is suggested [33]. The American Gastroenterological Association Institute Technical Review recommended follow-up by EUS or endoscopy at regular intervals for gastric SETs smaller than 3 cm [34]. However, in 2010, the National Comprehensive Cancer Network has recommended surgical resection of GISTs larger than 2 cm because of their malignant potential [35]. Lesions involving the muscularis propria are usually removed surgically because the complete endoscopic resection of these lesions is associated with the risk of perforation [36]. Endoscopic resection of gastric SETs from the muscularis propria (well-margined, endoluminal growth, 2–5 cm in size), results in complete endoscopic resection in 64% of cases [37].

3. EUS compared to other imaging modalities

Usually US, CT, and MRI are not sensitive enough to detect and characterize smaller SELs. Often it is impossible to differentiate them by endoscopy alone. EUS provides diagnostic information only for very large SELs. Like CT and MRI, it can also provide useful information on perigastric structures and when malignancy and metastasis is suspected. The diagnostic accuracy of MDCT is expected to be improved to even higher levels. Overall accuracy of MDCT in detection of SELs from a recent study was 78.8–85.3% [38], EUS has a history of higher accuracy in detecting and assessing the size and location of SELs comparison to other radiological imaging modalities. The narrow differential diagnosis of SELs afforded by the use of EUS is more effective than when the decision between observations with surveillance in patients with suspected benign lesions or resection when the lesion is likely to be malignant is taken (**Table 2**). In the differentiation between SELs and extraluminal compression, EUS also demonstrates a higher accuracy than endoscopy, ultrasonography, and CT. It has been reported that US and CT established the diagnosis in only 16% of cases, compared with 100% for EUS. In another comparison study of US, CT and EUS reported an accuracy of 22, 28, and 100%, respectively, in differentiating subepithelial tumors from extraluminal compression [39].

1	Endoscopy
2	Imaging (US, CT, MRI)
3	EUS with or without tissue acquisition
4	Further observation and surveillance for benign lesions
5	Endoscopic vs. surgical resection for premalignant and malignant lesions

Table 2. The practical approach.

4. Extramural lesions

When EUS demonstrates the integrity of all gut wall layers between the gut lumen and the lesion, it is safe to say that the lesion is an impression caused by an extramural structure. A normal spleen or splenic hilum is the most common etiology for SELs found to be of extramural origin [40]. Other normal anatomic variants such as the left lobe of the liver, the gallbladder, the pancreas tail, and enlarged lymph nodes can also sometimes be interpreted as SELs [41]. Adjacent structures, such as the aortic arch and vertebrae and enlarged lymph nodes can also press on the esophagus. Abnormal structures such as pancreatic pseudocysts, splenic artery aneurysm, aortic aneurysm, cystic tumor of the pancreas or liver, colonic tumors, and lymphoma [42] may also be interpreted as SELs. When using EUS, at a low frequency of 7.5 MHz, the examiner should survey the gross relationship between the extramural structure and the gut wall. Then, at a higher frequency of 12 MHz, the outer hyper-echoic serosal layer should be observed carefully to determine whether it is intact or disrupted. EUS is very sensitive to the identification of these extramural lesions. It has been reported that 11% of these were due to pathologic lesions, while others were related to adjacent normal organs or vessels [43].

5. Intramural lesions

5.1. Gastrointestinal stromal tumors (GIST)

GIST lesions originate from the muscular propria, which is the fourth layer, and specifically from the interstitial cell of Cajal. The pathophysiology of GIST as result of mutation in the KIT gene which codes for the c-Kit protein, a tyrosine kinase receptor and in nearly immunohistochemical 95% positive of CD117 (corresponds to c-kit activation, epitope of kit protein), and, sometimes, CD34 but negative for desmin. Leiomyomas express smooth muscle actin and desmin, and schwannomas produce S-100 protein [42, 44]. Approximately 80% of GI mesenchymal tumors are GISTs, and approximately 10–30% of GISTs are malignant. GIST lesions have the potential for malignant transformation and distant metastases. GIST appeared on endoscopy as submucosal lesions (**Figure 1A, B, E**). On EUS (**Figure 1C, D**), a GIST is typically a well-circumscribed, hypoechoic, relatively homogeneous mass that can arise from either the second hypoechoic layer (muscularis mucosa) or more frequently the fourth hypoechoic layer (muscularis propria). In addition to size and mucosal ulcer, other EUS characteristics have been considered as possible predictive factors, but size is the only consistently definitive predictive factor [45–48]. One study suggested that GISTs have a marginal hypoechoic halo and relatively higher echogenicity compared with the adjacent muscular layer [49]. Another study reported that the internal hypoechoic feature could be suggested as a predictive marker of tumor progression [47]. The presence of two of these three features had a positive predictive value of 100% for malignant or borderline-malignant tumors [50]. A multicenter study reported that malignancy or indeterminate GIST status correlated with the presence of ulceration, tumor size larger than 3 cm, irregular margins, and gastric location, but not with hyperechoic or hypoechoic internal foci [51]. With hyper-enhanced GIST after infusion of ultrasound contrast, in consequence, the contrast-enhanced harmonic EUS (CEH-EUS) signal intensity of GIST is higher than other benign lesions [52]. In addition, another study reported that prediction of malignant GIST was possible with CEH-EUS by identifying intratumoral irregular vessels with 83% accuracy [63]. EUS-guided fine-needle aspiration (EUS-FNA) and EUS-guided biopsy (EUS) can be performed for immunohistochemical examination to achieve better diagnostic accuracy of GIST [53–62]. Risk of malignancy depends on the size, the number of cells at pathological evaluation and location (**Table 3**) If the lesion <2 cm and the mitotic count less than 5/50 HPF, the risk of malignancy is very low. A GIST larger 5 cm, 10/50 HPF and small bowel have a much higher risk [3, 40, 72, 73]. Pathologists classify GISTs as "very low risk," "low risk," "intermediate risk," and "high risk" according to the size of the mass and the mitotic count of the resected specimen [50, 63, 64]. Management of the case depends on the size and present symptoms. A lesion of more than 1 cm needs more evaluation, EUS, FNA, and FNB or additional surgical specimens. Because small (<1 cm), asymptomatic mesenchymal tumors are rarely malignant, a close follow-up with EUS may be justified. Referral to a medical oncologist is preferable before surgical resection to consider adjuvant therapy with Imatinib (Gleevec) for high risk lesions.

Excision is advised when growth of the lesion, a change in the echo pattern, or necrosis is noted during yearly follow-up with EUS. Surgical treatment is indicated for lesions >3 cm in diameter, with features suggestive of malignancy (**Table 4**). For lesions between 1 and 3 cm,

http://dx.doi.org/10.5772/67102

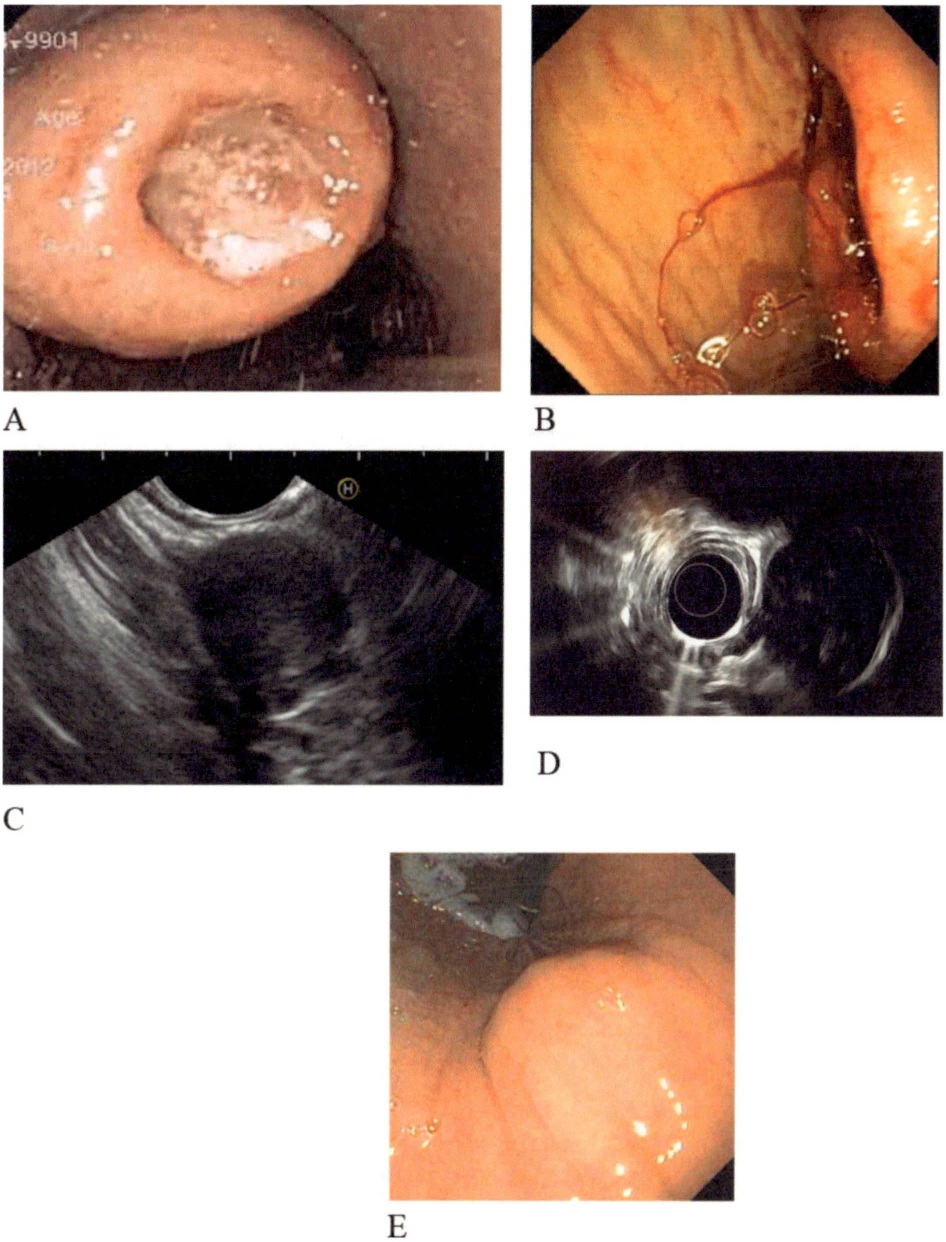

Figure 1. GIST: (A, B) Endoscopy shows an ulcerated submucosal lesion in the stomach. (C) EUS image showing homogeneous hypoechoic lesion. The lesion is located with the fourth layer, corresponding to the muscularis propria. (D) Malignant gastrointestinal stromal tumor (GIST) of the stomach. (E) Endoscopy view of small smooth submucosal mass noted in the rectum.

EUS-FNA can be recommended, or ESD can be chosen as a definite diagnostic and therapeutic tool with some risk of bleeding and perforation (2 to 3% in specialized centers). When the lesion is confirmed to be a GIST, the risk of malignant transformation needs to be discussed with the patient; more careful follow-up or early resection should then be considered.

History of iron–deficiency anemia
Ulcerated GIST
Stigmata of recent bleeding
Small bowel (jejunum or ileum)
Lesion larger than 2 cm
If the lesion is noted to be growing during the surveillance period

Table 3. GIST, indication of surgery.

Pathology	Muscularis mucosa	Submucosa	Muscularis propria	Serosa
GIST	X		XXX	
Leiomyoma	X		XX	
Pancreatic rest		XXX		
Carcinoid tumor	X	XXX		
Duplication cyst		XXX	X	
Granular cell tumor		XX		
Varices		XXX		

Table 4. Lists of the most common types of subepithelial lesions.

5.2. Leiomyoma

A leiomyoma is a benign tumor originating from the muscular layers (muscularis propria and muscularis mucosa) composed of well-differentiated smooth muscle cells with positive immunihistochemical findings for desmin and a smooth muscle action protein and negative CD117, CD34, and s100. Leiomyomas arise from muscularis mucosa more frequently than do GISTs. True leiomyomas are more commonly found in the esophagus and the small intestine but have been found throughout the GI tract. They rarely occur in the stomach or small bowel. In contrast, GISTs are rare in the esophagus and are more common in the stomach [65]. The risk of malignant transformation is very rare [3]. They appear by EUS as hypoechoic well-circumscribed masses in the muscularis propria or the muscularis mucosae (the fourth and second EUS layers, respectively). The approach and management of these depends on the size of the lesion. A lesion more than 1 cm in size should be referred to EUS for further evaluation. With a lesion <1 cm, annual surveillance with EGD or EUS every 1–2 years should take place if the patient is asymptomatic [66]. Leiomyomas appearing similar to GIST on EUS require tissue sampling with both histologic and immunohistochemical analysis for better diagnosis. The indication of surgical resection symptomatic (bleeding) and if the lesion is noted to be growing and enlarged with structural changes during the surveillance period (**Table 5**).

Risk of malignancy	Size	Mitotic count
Very low	<2 cm	<5/50 HPF
Low	2–5 cm	<5/50 HPF
Moderate	<5 cm	6–10/50 HPF
	>5 cm	<5/50 HPF
High	>5 cm	6—10/50 HPF
	Any size	>10/50 HPF

Table 5. Association between risk of malignancy and size and mitotic count.

5.3. Lipoma

Lipomas are common benign tumors composed of mature lipocytes, slow growing fatty tumors SELs that originate from the submucosal layer (third layer). They are found incidentally in any part of the GI tract, but more often in the gastric antrum than in the small bowel and can be seen more frequently in the lower tract [67, 68]. Endoscopically, most lipomas are soft solitary, with a smooth bulge and a yellow hue appearance (**Figure 2A, B**). They are indented when pressed with closed biopsy forceps (pillow or cushion sign) an indication highly specific for lipoma with specificity of 98% and low sensitivity of 40% were reported. On EUS (**Figure 2C, D, E**), lipomas characteristically appear as intensely hyperechoic, well circumscribed homogeneous lesions with clean regular margins arising from the third layer of the GI tract, which corresponds to the submucosa. The characteristic appearance on EUS is diagnostic and no further evaluation, including biopsy, is indicated [69, 70]. The endoscopic and EUS characteristics make it possible to diagnose lipoma in most cases.

Since there is no malignant potential, those lesions, they do not require biopsy or surgical resection or even regular endoscopic surveillance. Jumbo biopsy when performed often reveals nothing more than yellowish adipose tissue [71]. Once a lipoma has been confirmed, follow-up EUS is not recommended. Extremely rare lipomas can become ulcerated [40, 72]. Local excision is then advised for these symptomatic lipomas when associated with bleeding or obstruction. Resection is also recommended when it is impossible to distinguish between a lipoma and a malignant neoplasm, such as a liposarcoma, even though this lesion is rare in the GI tract [73].

5.4. Granular cell tumor

Granular cell tumors (GCT) are rare benign lesions of neural derivation thought to arise from Schwann cells as supported by immunophenotypic and ultrastructural evidence. Granular cell tumors are SELs usually originated from submucosal layer of GI tract and arise from Schwann cell. There are reports of malignant transformation in 2–3% of cases. De Ceglie et al. [74] the tumor grows towards the mucosal layer. Approximately 2.7–8.1% of GCTs involve the digestive tract, and these tumors are multiple in 5–12% of patients, they are usually found incidentally during endoscopy or colonoscopy and are located mostly in the esophagus; other locations

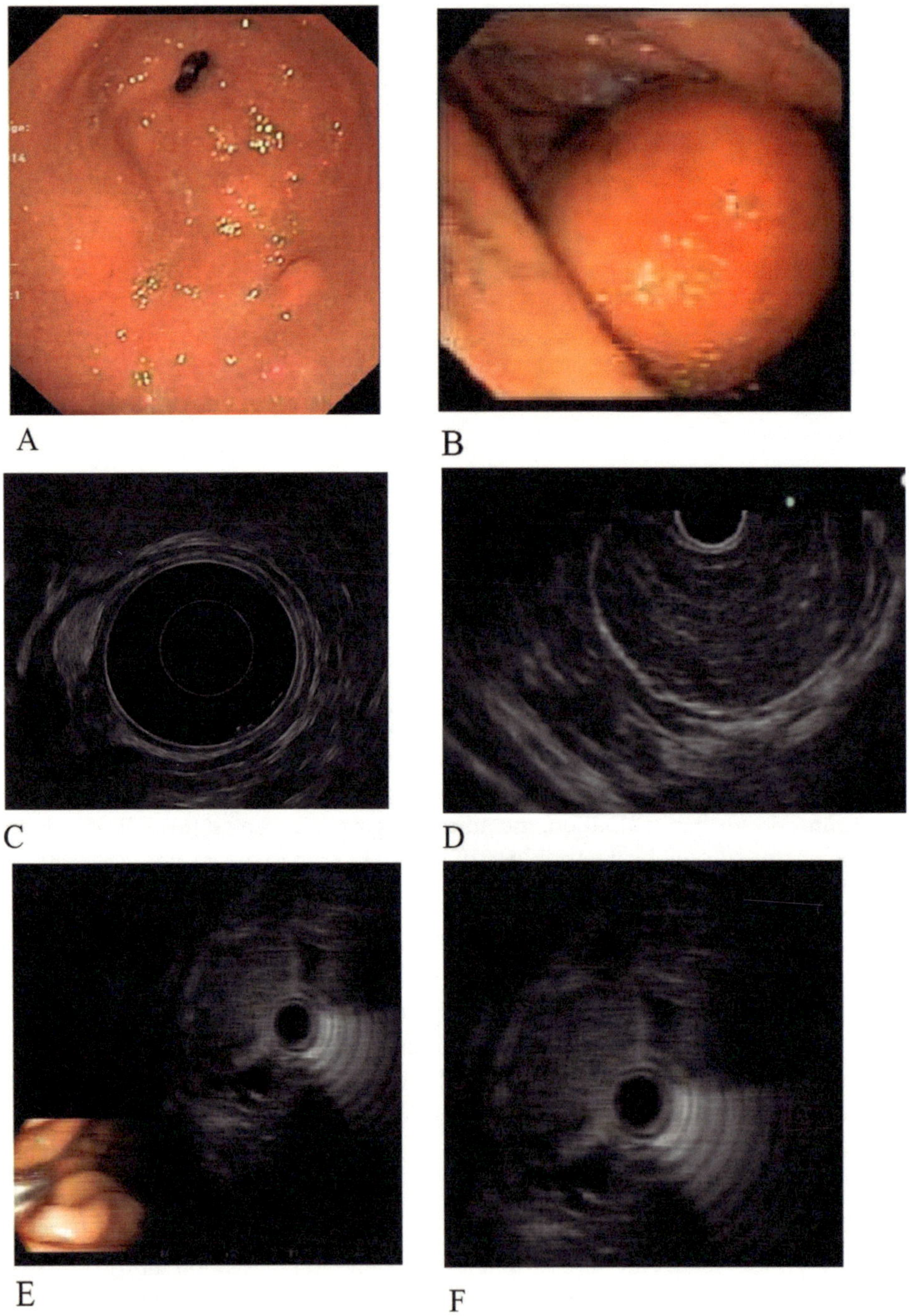

Figure 2. Lipoma. (A) Endoscopic view of a small elevated lesion covered with normal mucosa in the stomach. (B) Endoscopic view of a large elevated lesion covered with normal mucosa in the duodenum. (C) EUS reveals a homogeneous, hyperechoic lesion with smooth borders within the third gastric wall layer. (D) EUS image showed a heterogeneous, hyperchoic lesion within the third layer of the duodenal wall layer. (E) EUS reveals a large hyperechoic raised from the third colonic wall layer.

http://dx.doi.org/10.5772/67102

include the stomach (10%) and rarely the colon or rectum. Endoscopically, they appear as small firm, isolated nodules or polyps resembling molar teeth, with normal overlying mucosa having a yellow hue (**Figure 3A**). On EUS (**Figure 3B**), GCTs appear as hypoechoic, homogeneous lesions with smooth margins originating from the second or third layer of the GI tract, which corresponds to deep mucosa or submucosa. Mucosal biopsy using a regular forceps is usually helpful. The risk of malignancy is low, but the size of the tumor is an important factor. Lesions >4 cm increase the risk to around 2–4% [2]. Cytologic or histopathologic evaluation staining for S-100 can be helpful in differentiating this tumor [75]. For asymptomatic GCTs that are not excised, surveillance with EUS every 1–2 years is recommended to monitor changes in size. Local endoscopic snare excision can be performed for small tumors limited to the mucosa (**Figure 3C**).

5.5. Ectopic pancreas

Heterotopic pancreas tissue (aberrant pancreas or ectopic pancreatic tissue)—these terms are used to describe ectopic pancreatic tissue lying outside its normal location with no anatomic or vascular connection to the pancreas proper. They are typically discovered incidentally during endoscopy, surgery, or autopsy, in approximately 1 of every 500 operations performed in the

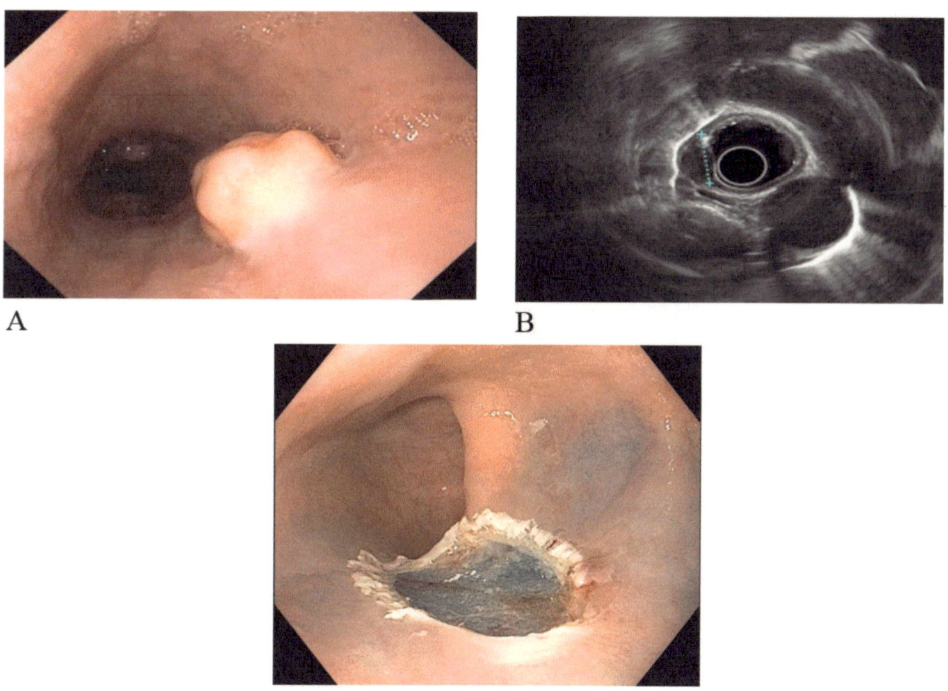

Figure 3. Granular cell tumor (GCT) of the esophagus. (A) Small, round, molar tooth-like, polypoid lesion in the esophagus. (B) Endosonographic image revealed a homogeneous, hypoechoic lesion with smooth margins is noted within the fourth layer. (C) Endoscopic image showed a EMR defect of GCT.

upper abdomen. The incidence in autopsy series has been estimated to be between 1 and 2% and in some reported autopsy series up to 13.7%. About 90% of the lesions are located within the stomach, and mainly in the gastric antrum, the duodenum, the small intestine, or anywhere in the GI tract. Most often asymptomatic incidental findings on endoscopy, they have been reported to present with nausea, epigastric pain, weight loss, hematemesis, ulceration, bleeding, acute pancreatitis and, rarely, gastric cyst formation, outlet obstruction, obstructive jaundice, dysphagia, and malignancy [76, 77]. These lesions have essentially no malignant potential, but there are rare case reports of adenocarcinoma arising from ectopic tissue [78].

Endoscopically (**Figure 4A, B**), this will typically be a small nodule with a central area of umbilication at the center of the lesion that corresponds to a draining duct. On deep biopsy sampling histologically, the presence of pancreatic acinar tissue will confirm the diagnosis. On EUS (**Figure 4C, D**) evaluation, it will have a heterogeneous hypoechoic. EUS features are heterogeneous

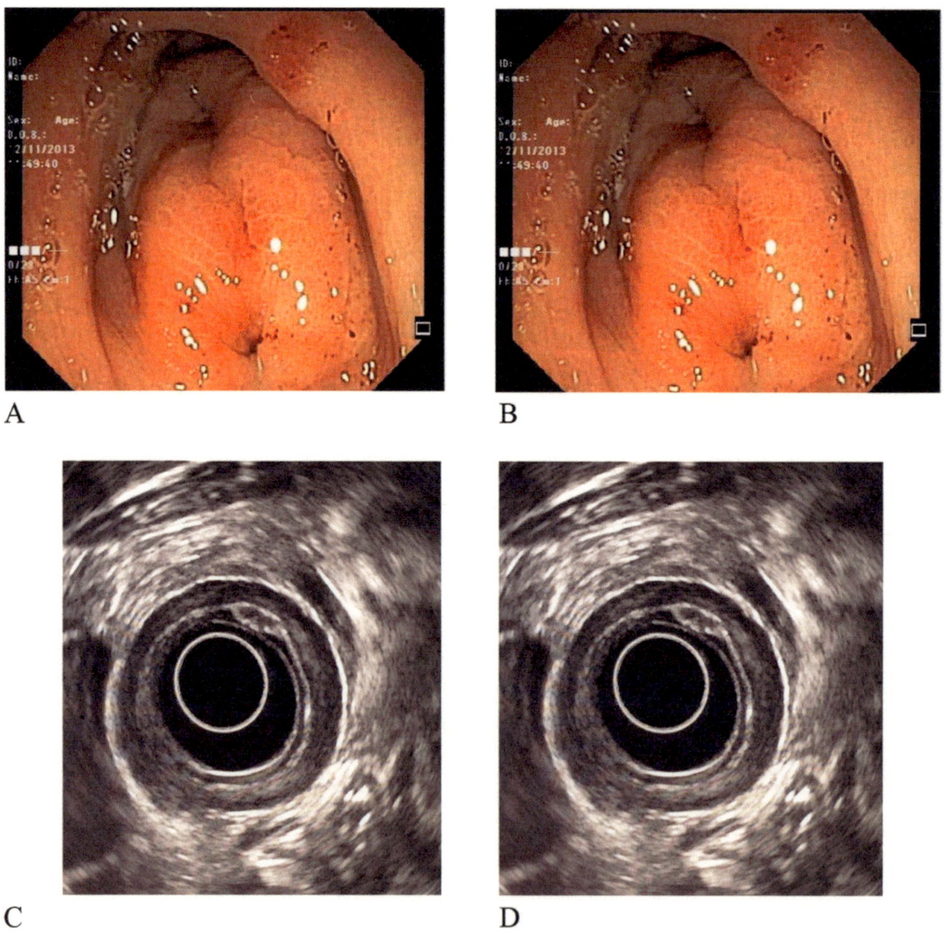

Figure 4. Pancreatic rest: (A and B) Endoscopic image of atypical raised submucosal lesion in the gastric antrum. A large umblicated lesion, resembling diffused mucosal lesion (C and D), EUS image (different patient) showing a well defined, hypoechoic lesion involving the third gastric layers.

lesions, mainly hypoechoic or intermediate echogenic lesions located within the submucosal layer (the third EUS layer) accompanied by scattered small hyperechoic areas. Generally, an anechoic area and fourth layer thickening will accompany the lesions. Anechoic cystic or tubular structures within the lesion correlate with ductal structures. However, these lesions may develop in any location from the deep mucosal to the serosal layer. The management of aberrant pancreas tissue remains controversial. It should be guided by the symptoms and the possibility of malignancy. Asymptomatic lesions do not necessarily require resection and can simply be followed up. If there are severe symptoms removal is advised. Endoscopic removal is useful both for accurate diagnosis and treatment, although surgical resection is preferred to endoscopic resection when the muscularis propria is involved [79]. Cap-assisted endoscopic mucosal resection is an effective manner of obtaining adequate tissue for histologic diagnosis and management [80].

5.6. Carcinoid tumor

Carcinoid tumors are slow-growing neuroendocrine tumors arising from entero-chromaffin-like (ECL) cells with malignant potential. They may arise at various sites anywhere in the GI tract, most commonly the GI tract and lung. GI carcinoid tumors are generally discovered incidentally during endoscopy, surgery, or autopsy from the appendix, rectum, stomach, and small intestine, and at least 25% of all carcinoid tumors occur within the small bowel (ileum, followed by the jejunum, and then the duodenum). The gastric carcinoid tumors account for 9% of all carcinoid tumors [81, 82]. Rectal carcinoids are common and represent approximately 20% of all GI carcinoid lesions. Female patients predominate. Carcinoid tumors from different areas of the GI tract will have potentially varying presentation and symptoms. Carcinoid tumors are usually asymptomatic, but rare complications include hemorrhage, abdominal pain, intestinal obstruction, and the endocrine carcinoid syndrome that results from the secretion of functionally active substances. Endoscopically (**Figure 5A, B**), carcinoid tumors appear as small, round, sessile, or polypoid lesions with a smooth surface and a yellow hue. They usually have normal overlying mucosa and seldom ulcerate. Gastric and ileal carcinoids are commonly multiple, whereas those arising elsewhere are typically solitary. Deep mucosal biopsy is normally diagnostic. EUS (**Figure 5C, D, E**) appearance of carcinoids is usually that of a homogeneous, well demarcated, and mildly hypoechoic or isoechoic mass. These lesions arise from the second layer of the GI tract and may invade beyond the third submucosal layer. Usually originating from the deep mucosal layer and penetrating into the submucosal layer, they may have the classic "salt and pepper" pattern. EUS accurately defines the size and extent of these masses and can guide management. When the lesion is smaller than 2 cm, does not invade further than the third layer, and no adenopathy is noted, endoscopic resection is possible [83, 84] (**Figure 5F**, **Table 6**).

5.7. Rectal carcinoid tumors

Rectal carcinoid tumors are frequently discovered during routine screening by colonoscopy. The size of the lesion is a key factor in risk for metastasis. Lesions <1 cm have rarely metastasized, and endoscopic resection is potentially curative [85, 86]. Small lesions of <1 cm in size that are confined to the submucosa should be removed endoscopically. Larger lesions (>2 cm), or lesions with penetration into the muscularis propria layer on EUS, or lesions with enlarged regional lymphadenopathy should be referred for surgical resection [87, 88].

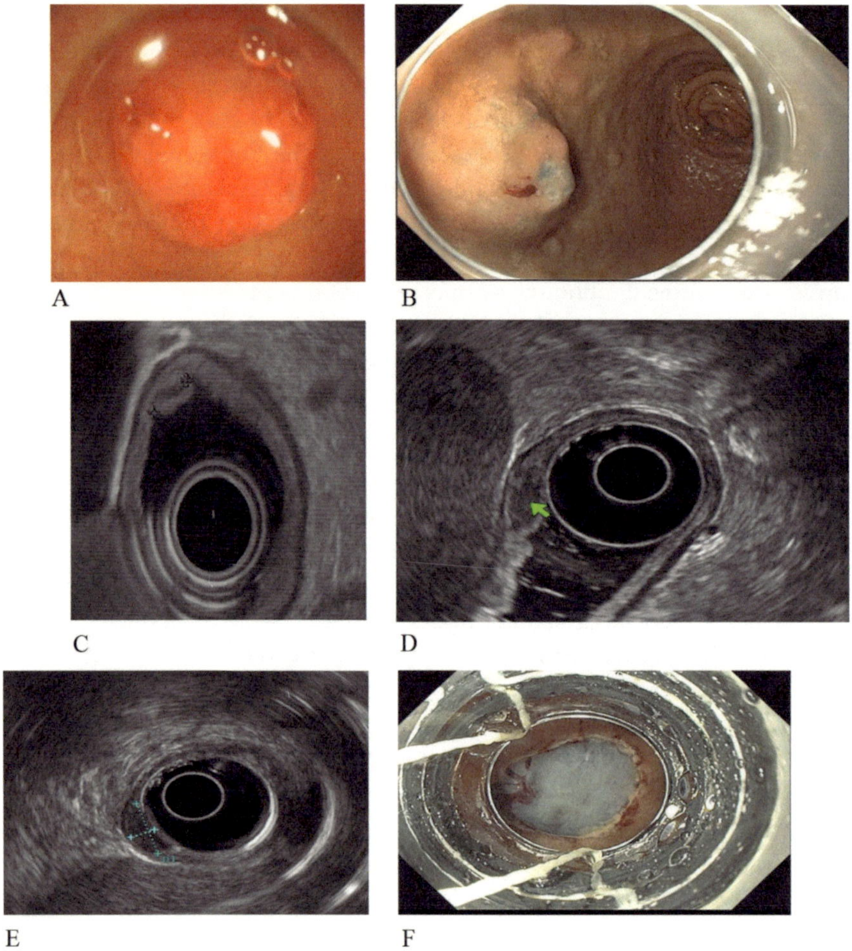

Figure 5. Carcinoid tumor. (A and B) Endoscopic images of a round submucosal lesion in the stomach and duodenal, respectively. (C -E) Endosonographic views of a homogeneous, hypoechoic lesions were located in the gastric and duodenum within the third layer, corresponding to the submucoal layer. (F) Endoscopy image of post-EMR of duodenal carcinoid.

Symptomatic (bleeding)
If the lesion is noted to be growing and enlarged with structural changes during the surveillance period

Table 6. Indication of surgical resection.

5.8. Varices

Here, we are talking mainly about gastric varices or those in other areas of the small bowel requiring EUS evaluation (**Figure 6A, B**), compared to esophageal varices, which are obvious by routine endoscopy [89]. Patient history and portal hypertensive gastropathy will usually support diagnoses of varices versus other etiologies of SELs. Gastric varices can be

http://dx.doi.org/10.5772/67102

misdiagnosed endoscopically as submucosal tumors or thickened gastric folds. EUS (**Figure 6C**) will reveal varices as small, round to oval, and anechoic structures or tubular hypoechoic or anechoic structure within the submucosa (the third EUS layer) that demonstrates venous flow when evaluated with Doppler. When gastric varices grow larger, they appear as anechoic, serpentine, tubular structures with smooth margins, accompanied by perigastric collateral vessels. In comparative studies, EUS was shown to be inferior to endoscopy for detecting and grading esophageal varices, but it permitted detection of fundic varices earlier and more often than endoscopy in patients with portal hypertension. EUS can be one of the interventional modalities of bleeding varices. EUS was used in the treatment of varices by making it possible to inject a sclerosing agent into perforating veins. EUS is used to guide cyanoacrylate injection and case reports of EUS-guided coiling of refractory bleeding varices. [90] Also, there is a report about transesophageal EUS-guided treatment of gastric fundic varices. This procedure was shown to be safe and successful in 96% of cases [91].

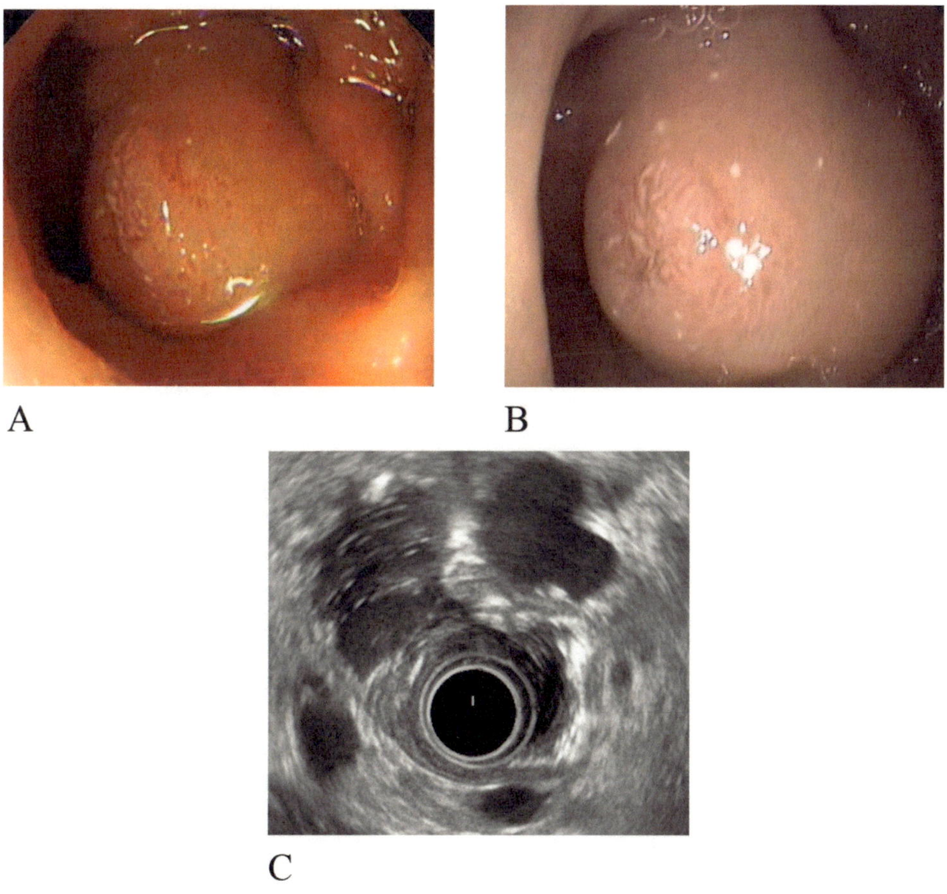

Figure 6. Ectopic duodenal varices. (A and B) Endoscopic views of a large bulging mass lesion at the duodenum. (C) EUS confirmed large, anechoic, tubular, submucosal vessels with multiple extramural collateral vascular structures.

5.9. Cyst and duplication cysts

Gastrointestinal duplication cysts are also identified throughout adulthood [92]. The cysts are benign lesions resulting from an error in the embryonic development of the foregut and can be found either within or adjacent to the wall of the gastrointestinal tract. The cysts can enlarge with secretions resulting in mass effect, infection, rupture, or bleeding [92]. The stomach is the least common site for GI duplication cysts but they can be anywhere in GI tract. On endoscopy appeared as small and smooth subepithelial lesion (**Figure 7A**) and EUS (**Figure 7B–D**), cysts in the GI tract appear as anechoic sharply demarcated structures, ounded, or ovoid structures with dorsal acoustic accentuation originating from the second and third layers. However, some may be seen as hypoechoic lesions containing echogenic foci. Cystic submucosal tumors can be classified into three EUS types (simple cystic, multicystic, and solid cystic tumors). Duplication cysts on EUS appear as anechoic, homogeneous lesions with regular margins arising from the third layer or extrinsic to the GI wall. The walls of duplication cysts may be seen as three or five layer structures because of the presence of the submucosa and the muscle layer [93]. Duplication cysts are believed to have a low malignant potential, but some case reports have described malignant transformation. Complications are rare and may include dysphagia,

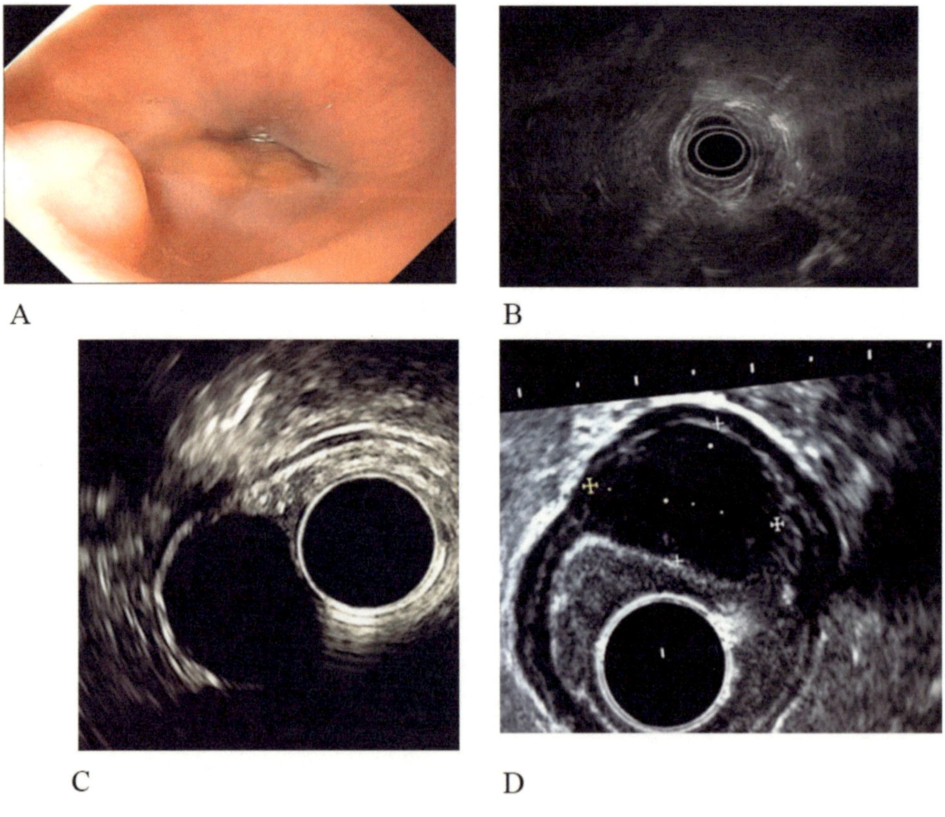

Figure 7. Esophageal and gastric cysts: (A) Endoscopic view of a small bulge at the mid-esophagus. (B) EUS revealed a well-demarcated, round, anechoic, within the third layer of esophageal wall. (C and D) EUS images revealed a sharply demarcated, anechoic, ovoid structure within the third gastric wall layer.

abdominal pain, bleeding, and pancreatitis when the cyst is located near the ampulla of Vater. Bronchogenic cysts represent 50–60% of all mediastinal cysts, and they can be diagnosed easily with EUS as anechoic mass without wall layers. EUS-FNA would cause serious complications, including cyst infection and mediastinitis. Antibiotic prophylaxis is therefore needed and close attention should be paid to avoid accidental instrumentation (**Tables 7–9**).

Lesion <1 cm	Annual EGD surveillance
Lesion 1–2 cm	Annual EGD surveillance vs. endoscopic resection if there is no deeper penetration to submucosal layer
Lesion >2 cm	Surgical resection

Table 7. Management approach [95].

Type I gastric carcinoid tumors are associated with atrophic gastritis, pernicious anemia and hypergastrinemia	Low malignant potential
Type II gastric carcinoid tumors are also associated with hypergastrinemia, but the high gastrin levels are due to Zollinger-Ellison syndrome or MEN-1 (multiple endocrine neoplasia syndrome, type 1)	Intermediate malignant potential
Type III gastric carcinoid tumors (normal gastrin levels) are the sporadic form	High malignant potential

Table 8. Gastric carcinoid tumors [115].

Type I and II	Endoscopic resection for small lesion, <1–2 cm
Type I and II	Surgical resection for large lesions >2 cm or Multiple lesions (>5) Antrectomy or fundectomy (removal of G-cell or ECL Surveillance every 6–12 months
Type III lesion (normal gastrin level)	Surgical resection with lymph node dissection

Table 9. Management of gastric carcinoid tumors.

5.10. Glomus tumors

A glomus tumor originates from smooth muscle cells of the glomus body and originates from modified vascular smooth muscle cells, and peripheral soft tissue, [94]. A glomus tumor of the gastrointestinal tract is a rare disease, and most of them are found in the stomach. The majority of gastric glomus tumors are benign and found incidentally as a SEL during routine endoscopy. However, some malignant gastric glomus tumors and cases of ulcerative bleeding have been reported. Contrast-enhanced CT reveals a homogeneous hyperdense enhancement on early and delayed phase. On evaluation by EUS, glomus tumors are shown as a circumscribed and hypoechoic mass internal heterogeneous echo mixed with hyperechogenic in the third or fourth layer [95]. Doppler signals suggest the hypervascularity of these lesions located in the submucosa and muscularis propria—also rarely in the serosa (third, fourth, and fifth EUS layers, respectively). Fine-needle aspiration with cytologic and immunohistochemical staining positive for smooth muscle actin and vimentin and negative for CD117 help to differentiate this lesion [96].

5.11. Inflammatory fibroid polyps

Inflammatory fibroid polyp is a rare benign polypoid lesion that is usually found in the stomach, occasionally in the small bowel, and rarely in the esophagus or large bowel [97]. The lesion is located in the second or third layer of the gastric wall, with an intact fourth layer. Sometimes the internal echo pattern is heterogeneous or hyperechoic [98].

5.12. Lymphoma

Primary lymphomas of the GI tract are usually B-cell type lymphomas, including diffuse large B-cell, mantle cell, Burkitt's, and mucosa associated lymphoid tissue (MALT) [99]. Endoscopy with standard biopsies is often not enough for accurate diagnosis. On EUS, a gastrointestinal lymphoma usually appears as a hypoechoic lesion in the deep mucosa or submucosa (second or third EUS layer). EUS is of key importance for diagnosis with FNA cab being used for flow cytometry [100].

6. Histologic assessment of subepithelial lesions

When the SEL is ulcerated, careful biopsy provides an accurate diagnosis. However, for most SELs, the results of endoscopic biopsy are inconclusive [101]. Trials with a bite-on-bite technique have been undertaken [102, 103]. However, the sensitivity, specificity, and accuracy of cytological evaluations of intramural lesions are all lower than those for SELs in lymph nodes or organs adjacent to the GI tract. It has been reported that the sensitivity of EUS-FNA for mediastinal masses, mediastinal lymph nodes, celiac lymph nodes, pancreatic tumors, and submucosal tumors was 88, 81, 80, 75, and 60%, respectively [104–107]. Subsequent endoscopic resection procedures for these lesions will be difficult. EUS-guided tissue diagnosis is useful for patients with GIST who have metastasis (**Figure 8A, B**). In these studies, no significant difference in diagnostic accuracy was noted according to the size of the FNA needle, but the 25-G needle easily punctured small mobile SELs and the 19-G needle showed excellent differentiation between GIST and leiomyoma by enabling tissue procurement for immunohistochemical studies (**Figure 8C, D**). The average reported accuracy of EUS-FNA in the diagnosis of SELs lesions is approximately 80% [108–110]. The development of new EUS-FNB needles promises better GI SET diagnosis rates [111]. In some later prospective studies, however, the diagnostic yield of EUS-TCB in patients with gastric SELs was not better than that of EUS-FNA, and the tissue core obtained with EUS-TCB was not sufficient to examine for mitotic index in GIST. It is clear though that EUS-TCB can be complementary to EUS-FNA [112]. Complications of EUS-FNA and EUS-TCB are very rare, but can include infection, bleeding and perforation. The newly developed ProCore needle (Cook Endoscopy, Winston-Salem, NC, USA) or Side-Port needle (Olympus, Tokyo, Japan) both appear promising. Core biopsy along with aspiration material is made possible with these types of FNA needles [113]. It is important to note that any form of needle biopsy carries the possibility of sampling error, and a negative finding does not exclude malignancy in GISTs. This diagnostic method should be considered for SETs before determining whether tumors should undergo long-term monitoring or surgical resection.

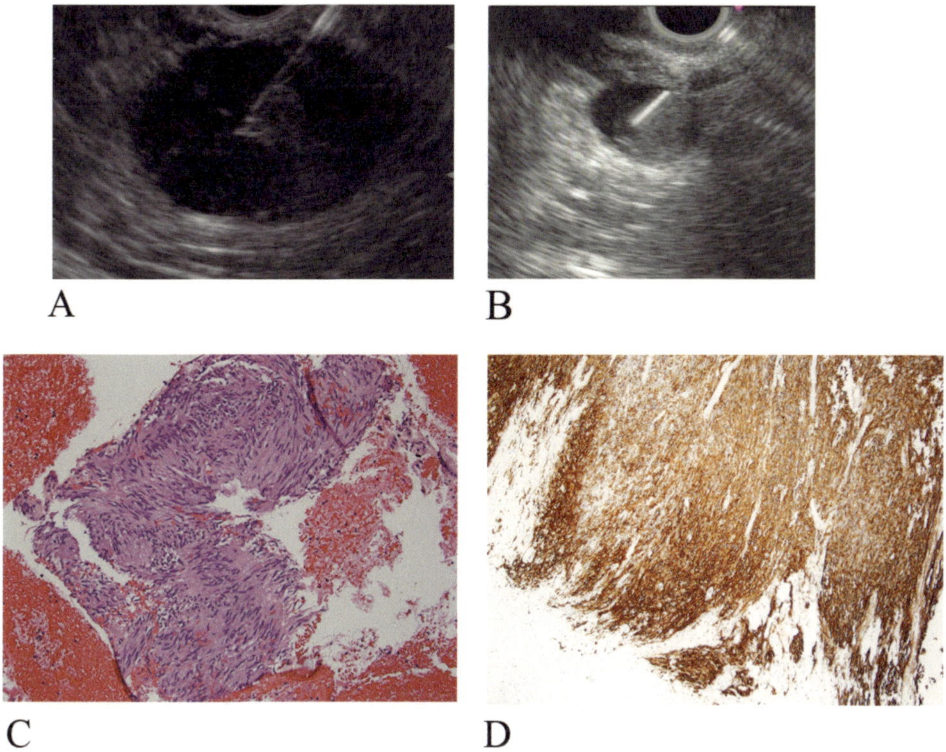

Figure 8. EUS-FNA of a gastric and rectal GIST. (A and B) FNA needle was inserted into the mass and the stylet was removed as the needle was moved back and forth within the lesion. (C) Slide reveled H&E 20× Spindle Cell Neoplasm. (D) Immunohistochemical stains show a positive reaction of the tumor cells for smooth muscle actin and positive of C-KIT.

7. Management of subepithelial lesions

Management of SELs can be guided by EUS findings. Extraluminal compression by adjacent organs and benign submucosal lesions such as lipomas or simple cysts do not need further treatment or follow-up. Pancreatic rest and inflammatory fibroid polyps can be followed in situ. Suspicious lesions, such as carcinoid tumors, can be diagnosed with endoscopic biopsy. Biopsy should be avoided in lesions that are suspected varices. For deeply located hypoechoic lesions, EUS-FNA, or EUS-TCB can be performed for tissue diagnosis. If resection is planned, ESD can be used as a therapeutic tool for small mass lesions arising from the submucosal or inner circular muscularis propria layer, instead of surgical resection. Surveillance may be appropriate for SELs without definite tissue diagnosis in patients who are at high operative risk. If the lesion is a suspected GIST, changes in size and echogenicity should be monitored. If the size increases or malignant features (echogenic foci, heterogeneity, internal cystic space, irregularity of extraluminal margins, and adjacent lymphadenopathy) develop, resection should be recommended. The follow-up interval depends on the index of suspicion of the examiner and is usually 1 year. When the characteristics of the lesion do not change on two consecutive follow-up examinations with EUS, a longer follow-up interval may be justified [40, 114, 115].

8. Summary

The most common SELs have all been discussed in this chapter. Their characteristics have been summarized and the appropriate diagnostic techniques, therapeutic modalities and immunohistochemical markers used to help in their identification have been reviewed. Most SELs should be referred for EUS evaluation especially if the SEL is more than 1 cm in size. Based on the specific EUS outcomes, majority of the cases a presumptive diagnosis can be made. It is the best test to help and plays an important role in directing further diagnosis and management. EUS-FNA is a good method for tissue diagnosis when a GI SET is suspected. Cytological examination with IHS is essential for the best diagnostic performance in GI SETs. EUS-TCB is good for tissue acquisition, but is associated with some technical challenges. EUS is also plays a major role in endoscopic resection because it can enable the examiner to determine the depth and originating wall layer of the lesion. EUS can also be used in the follow-up lesion if it is not resected.

Author details

Abed Al-Lehibi[1*] and Khaled Bamakhrama[2]

*Address all correspondence to: aha0021@gmail.com

1 Gastroenterology and Hepatology Division, King Saud Bin Abdulaziz University-Health Science, Saudi Arabia

2 Dubai Medical College, Rashid Hospital, Dubai, UAE

References

[1] Hedenbro JL, Ekelund M, Wetterberg P. Endoscopic diagnosis of submucosal gastric lesions. The results after routine endoscopy. Surg Endosc. 1991;5(1):20–3.

[2] Polkowski M. Endoscopic ultrasound and endoscopic ultrasound-guided fine-needle biopsy for the diagnosis of malignant submucosal tumors. Endoscopy. 2005;37(7):635–45.

[3] Humphris JL, Jones DB. Subepithelial mass lesions in the upper gastrointestinal tract. J Gastroenterol Hepatol. 2008 Apr;23(4):556–66.

[4] Silberhumer GR, Hufschmid M, Wrba F, Gyoeri G, Schoppmann S, Tribl B, Wenzl E, Prager G, Laengle F, Zacherl J. Surgery for gastrointestinal stromal tumors of the stomach. J Gastrointest Surg. 2009;13(7):1213–9.

[5] Park YS, Park SW, Kim TI, Song SY, Choi EH, Chung JB, Kang JK. Endoscopic enucleation of upper-GI submucosal tumors by using an insulated-tip electrosurgical knife. Gastrointest Endosc. 2004;59(3):409–15.

[6] Moon JS. Endoscopic ultrasound-guided fine needle aspiration in submucosal lesion. Clin Endosc. 2012;45(2):117–23.

[7] Sakamoto H, Kitano M, Kudo M. Diagnosis of subepithelial tumors in the upper gastrointestinal tract by endoscopic ultrasonography. World J Radiol. 2010,28;2(8):289–97.

[8] Kim GH, Cho YK, Kim EY, Kim HK, Cho JW, Lee TH, Moon JS; Korean EUS Study Group Comparison of 22-gauge aspiration needle with 22-gauge biopsy needle in endoscopic ultrasonography-guided subepithelial tumor sampling. Scand J Gastroenterol. 2014;49(3):347–54.

[9] Landi B, Palazzo L. The role of endosonography in submucosal tumours. Best Pract Res Clin Gastroenterol. 2009;23(5):679–701.

[10] Tae HJ, Lee HL, Lee KN, Jun DW, Lee OY, Han DS, Yoon BC, Choi HS, Hahm JS. Deep biopsy via endoscopic submucosal dissection in upper gastrointestinal subepithelial tumors: a prospective study. Endoscopy. 2014;46(10):845–50.

[11] Ji JS, Lee BI, Choi KY, Kim BW, Choi H, Huh M, Chung WC, Chae HS, Chung IS. Diagnostic yield of tissue sampling using a bite-on-bite technique for incidental subepithelial lesions. Korean J Intern Med. 2009;24(2):101–5.

[12] Lee S, Seo DW, Choi JH, Park do H, Lee SS, Lee SK, Kim MH. Evaluation of the feasibility and efficacy of forward-viewing endoscopic ultrasound. Gut Liver. 2015,23;9(5):679–84.

[13] Nesje LB, Laerum OD, Svanes K, Ødegaard S. Subepithelial masses of the gastrointestinal tract evaluated by endoscopic ultrasonography. Eur J Ultrasound. 2002;15(1–2):45–54.

[14] Chak A. EUS in submucosal tumors. Gastrointest Endosc. 2002;56(4 Suppl):S43–8.

[15] Nguyen-Tang T, Shah JN, Sanchez-Yague A, Binmoeller KF. Use of the front-view forward-array echoendoscope to evaluate right colonic subepithelial lesions. Gastrointest Endosc. 2010;72(3):606–10.

[16] Reddymasu SC, Oropeza-Vail M, Pakseresht K, Moloney B, Esfandyari T, Grisolano S, Buckles D, Olyaee M. Are endoscopic ultrasonography imaging characteristics reliable for the diagnosis of small upper gastrointestinal subepithelial lesions? J Clin Gastroenterol. 2012;46(1):42–5.

[17] Karaca C, Turner BG, Cizginer S, Forcione D, Brugge W. Accuracy of EUS in the evaluation of small gastric subepithelial lesions. Gastrointest Endosc. 2010;71(4):722–7.

[18] Ji F, Wang ZW, Wang LJ, Ning JW, Xu GQ. Clinicopathological characteristics of gastrointestinal mesenchymal tumors and diagnostic value of endoscopic ultrasonography. J Gastroenterol Hepatol. 2008;23(8 Pt 2): e318–24.

[19] Kwon JG, Kim EY, Kim YS, Chun JW, Chung JT, You SS, Ha HK, Lee CH, Kim HG, Cho CH. [Accuracy of endoscopic ultrasonographic impression compared with pathologic diagnosis in gastrointestinal submucosal tumors]. Korean J Gastroenterol. 2005;45(2):88–96.

[20] Akahoshi K, Sumida Y, Matsui N, Oya M, Akinaga R, Kubokawa M, Motomura Y, Honda K, Watanabe M, Nagaie T. Preoperative diagnosis of gastrointestinal stromal tumor by endoscopic ultrasound-guided fine needle aspiration. World J Gastroenterol. 2007,14;13(14):2077–82.

[21] Polkowski M, Gerke W, Jarosz D, Nasierowska-Guttmejer A, Rutkowski P, Nowecki ZI, Ruka W, Regula J, Butruk E. Diagnostic yield and safety of endoscopic ultrasound-guided trucut [corrected] biopsy in patients with gastric submucosal tumors: a prospective study. Endoscopy. 2009;41(4):329–34.

[22] Chen VK, Eloubeidi MA. Endoscopic ultrasound-guided fine-needle aspiration of intramural and extraintestinal mass lesions: diagnostic accuracy, complication assessment, and impact on management. Endoscopy. 2005;37(10):984–9.

[23] Demetri GD, von Mehren M, Antonescu CR, DeMatteo RP, Ganjoo KN, Maki RG, Pisters PW, Raut CP, Riedel RF, Schuetze S, Sundar HM, Trent JC, Wayne JD. NCCN Task Force report: update on the management of patients with gastrointestinal stromal tumors. J Natl Compr Canc Netw. 2010;8(Suppl 2):S1–41.

[24] Ando N, Goto H, Niwa Y, Hirooka Y, Ohmiya N, Nagasaka T, Hayakawa T. The diagnosis of GI stromal tumors with EUS-guided fine needle aspiration with immunohistochemical analysis. Gastrointest Endosc. 2002;55(1):37–43.

[25] Kida M, Araki M, Miyazawa S, Ikeda H, Takezawa M, Kikuchi H, Watanabe M, Imaizumi H, Koizumi W. Comparison of diagnostic accuracy of endoscopic ultrasound-guided fine-needle aspiration with 22- and 25-gauge needles in the same patients. J Interv Gastroenterol. 2011;1(3):102–107.

[26] Varadarajulu S, Bang JY, Hebert-Magee S. Assessment of the technical performance of the flexible 19-gauge EUS-FNA needle. Gastrointest Endosc. 2012;76(2):336–43.

[27] Polkowski M, Larghi A, Weynand B, Boustière C, Giovannini M, Pujol B, Dumonceau JM, European Society of Gastrointestinal Endoscopy (ESGE). Learning, techniques, and complications of endoscopic ultrasound (EUS)-guided sampling in gastroenterology: European Society of Gastrointestinal Endoscopy (ESGE) Technical Guideline. Endoscopy. 2012;44(2):190–206.

[28] Storch I, Jorda M, Thurer R, Raez L, Rocha-Lima C, Vernon S, Ribeiro A. Advantage of EUS Trucut biopsy combined with fine-needle aspiration without immediate on-site cytopathologic examination. Gastrointest Endosc. 2006;64(4):505–11.

[29] Iglesias-Garcia J, Poley JW, Larghi A, Giovannini M, Petrone MC, Abdulkader I, Monges G, Costamagna G, Arcidiacono P, Biermann K, Rindi G, Bories E, Dogloni C, Bruno M, Dominguez-Muñoz JE. Feasibility and yield of a new EUS histology needle: results from a multicenter, pooled, cohort study. Gastrointest Endosc. 2011;73(6):1189–96.

[30] Shen EF, Arnott ID, Plevris J, Penman ID. Endoscopic ultrasonography in the diagnosis and management of suspected upper gastrointestinal submucosal tumours. Br J Surg. 2002;89(2):231–5.

[31] Goto O, Kambe H, Niimi K, Mochizuki S, Asada-Hirayama I, Minatsuki C, Ono S, Kodashima S, Yamamichi N, Yamaji Y, Fujishiro M, Koike K. Discrepancy in diagnosis of gastric submucosal tumor among esophagogastroduodenoscopy, CT, and endoscopic ultrasonography: a retrospective analysis of 93 consecutive cases. Abdom Imaging. 2012;37(6):1074–8.

[32] Hoteya S, Iizuka T, Kikuchi D, Yahagi N. Endoscopic submucosal dissection for gastric submucosal tumor, endoscopic sub-tumoral dissection. Dig Endosc. 2009;21(4):266–9.

[33] Seo SW, Hong SJ, Han JP, Choi MH, Song JY, Kim HK, Lee TH, Ko BM, Cho JY, Lee JS, Lee MS. Accuracy of a scoring system for the differential diagnosis of common gastric subepithelial tumors based on endoscopic ultrasonography. J Dig Dis. 2013;14(12):647–53.

[34] Hwang JH, Rulyak SD, Kimmey MB; American Gastroenterological Association Institute. American Gastroenterological Association Institute technical review on the management of gastric subepithelial masses. Gastroenterology. 2006;130(7):2217–28.

[35] Larghi A, Fuccio L, Chiarello G, Attili F, Vanella G, Paliani GB, Napoleone M, Rindi G, Larocca LM, Costamagna G, Ricci R. Fine-needle tissue acquisition from subepithelial lesions using a forward-viewing linear echoendoscope. Endoscopy. 2014;46(1):39–45.

[36] Menon L, Buscaglia JM. Endoscopic approach to subepithelial lesions. Ther Adv Gastroenterol. 2014;7(3):123–30.

[37] Hwang JC, Kim JH, Kim JH, Shin SJ, Cheong JY, Lee KM, Yoo BM, Lee KJ, Cho SW. Endoscopic resection for the treatment of gastric subepithelial tumors originated from the muscularis propria layer. Hepatogastroenterology. 2009;56(94–95):1281–6.

[38] Okten RS, Kacar S, Kucukay F, Sasmaz N, Cumhur T. Gastric subepithelial masses: evaluation of multidetector CT (multiplanar reconstruction and virtual gastroscopy) versus endoscopic ultrasonography. Abdom Imaging. 2012;37(4):519–30.

[39] Zhang QL, Nian WD. Endoscopic ultrasonography diagnosis in submucosal tumor of stomach. Endoscopy. 1998;30(Suppl 1):A69–71.

[40] Hwang JH, Saunders MD, Rulyak SJ, Shaw S, Nietsch H, Kimmey MB. A prospective study comparing endoscopy and EUS in the evaluation of GI subepithelial masses. Gastrointest Endosc. 2005;62(2):202–8.

[41] Rösch T, Kapfer B, Will U, Baronius W, Strobel M, Lorenz R, Ulm K; German EUS Club. Endoscopic ultrasonography. Accuracy of endoscopic ultrasonography in upper gastrointestinal submucosal lesions: a prospective multicenter study. Scand J Gastroenterol. 2002;37(7):856–62.

[42] Futagami K, Hata J, Haruma K, Yamashita N, Yoshida S, Tanaka S, Chayama K. Extracorporeal ultrasound is an effective diagnostic alternative to endoscopic ultrasound for gastric submucosal tumours. Scand J Gastroenterol. 2001;36(11):1222–6.

[43] Oztas E, Oguz D, Kurt M, Etik DO, Cicek B, Kekilli M, Onal IK, Sayilir A, Kacar S, Sahin B. Endosonographic evaluation of patients with suspected extraluminal compression or subepithelial lesions during upper gastrointestinal endoscopy. Eur J Gastroenterol Hepatol. 2011;23(7):586–92.

[44] Miettinen M, Sobin LH, Lasota J. Gastrointestinal stromal tumors of the stomach: a clinicopathologic, immunohistochemical, and molecular genetic study of 1765 cases with long-term follow-up. Am J Surg Pathol. 2005;29(1):52–68.

[45] Kim GH, Park DY, Kim S, Kim DH, Kim DH, Choi CW, Heo J, Song GA. Is it possible to differentiate gastric GISTs from gastric leiomyomas by EUS? World J Gastroenterol. 2009,21;15(27):3376–81.

[46] Jeon SW, Park YD, Chung YJ, Cho CM, Tak WY, Kweon YO, Kim SK, Choi YH. Gastrointestinal stromal tumors of the stomach: endosonographic differentiation in relation to histological risk. J Gastroenterol Hepatol. 2007;22(12):2069–75.

[47] Shah P, Gao F, Edmundowicz SA, Azar RR, Early DS. Predicting malignant potential of gastrointestinal stromal tumors using endoscopic ultrasound. Dig Dis Sci. 2009;54(6):1265–9.

[48] Onishi M, Tominaga K, Sugimori S, Machida H, Okazaki H, Yamagami H, Tanigawa T, Watanabe K, Watanabe T, Fujiwara Y, Arakawa T. Internal hypoechoic feature by EUS as a possible predictive marker for the enlargement potential of gastric GI stromal tumors. Gastrointest Endosc. 2012;75(4):731–8.

[49] Okai T, Minamoto T, Ohtsubo K, Minato H, Kurumaya H, Oda Y, Mai M, Sawabu N. Endosonographic evaluation of c-kit-positive gastrointestinal stromal tumor. Abdom Imaging. 2003;28(3):301–7.

[50] Palazzo L, Landi B, Cellier C, Cuillerier E, Roseau G, Barbier JP. Endosonographic features predictive of benign and malignant gastrointestinal stromal cell tumours. Gut. 2000;46(1):88–92.

[51] Nickl N. Decision analysis of hypoechoic intramural tumor study results. Gastrointest Endosc. 2002;56(suppl):S102.

[52] Kannengiesser K, Mahlke R, Petersen F, Peters A, Ross M, Kucharzik T, Maaser C. Contrast-enhanced harmonic endoscopic ultrasound is able to discriminate benign submucosal lesions from gastrointestinal stromal tumors. Scand J Gastroenterol. 2012;47(12):1515–20.

[53] Sakamoto H, Kitano M, Matsui S, Kamata K, Komaki T, Imai H, Dote K, Kudo M. Estimation of malignant potential of GI stromal tumors by contrast-enhanced harmonic EUS (with videos). Gastrointest Endosc. 2011;73(2):227–37.

[54] DeWitt J, Emerson RE, Sherman S, Al-Haddad M, McHenry L, Cote GA, Leblanc JK. Endoscopic ultrasound-guided Trucut biopsy of gastrointestinal mesenchymal tumor. Surg Endosc. 2011;25(7):2192–202.

[55] Watson RR, Binmoeller KF, Hamerski CM, Shergill AK, Shaw RE, Jaffee IM, Stewart L, Shah JN. Yield and performance characteristics of endoscopic ultrasound-guided fine needle aspiration for diagnosing upper GI tract stromal tumors. Dig Dis Sci. 2011;56(6):1757–62.

[56] Fernández-Esparrach G, Sendino O, Solé M, Pellisé M, Colomo L, Pardo A, Martínez-Pallí G, Argüello L, Bordas JM, Llach J, Ginès A. Endoscopic ultrasound-guided fine-needle aspiration and trucut biopsy in the diagnosis of gastric stromal tumors: a randomized crossover study. Endoscopy. 2010;42(4):292–9.

[57] Sepe PS, Moparty B, Pitman MB, Saltzman JR, Brugge WR. EUS-guided FNA for the diagnosis of GI stromal cell tumors: sensitivity and cytologic yield. Gastrointest Endosc. 2009;70(2):254–61.

[58] Chatzipantelis P, Salla C, Karoumpalis I, Apessou D, Sakellariou S, Doumani I, Papaliodi E, Konstantinou P. Endoscopic ultrasound-guided fine needle aspiration biopsy in the diagnosis of gastrointestinal stromal tumors of the stomach. A study of 17 cases. J Gastrointestin Liver Dis. 2008;17(1):15–20.

[59] Hizawa K, Matsumoto T, Kouzuki T, Suekane H, Esaki M, Fujishima M. Cystic submucosal tumors in the gastrointestinal tract: endosonographic findings and endoscopic removal. Endoscopy. 2000;32(9):712–4.

[60] Mochizuki Y, Kodera Y, Fujiwara M, Ito S, Yamamura Y, Sawaki A, Yamao K, Kato T. Laparoscopic wedge resection for gastrointestinal stromal tumors of the stomach: initial experience. Surg Today. 2006;36(4):341–7.

[61] Okubo K, Yamao K, Nakamura T, Tajika M, Sawaki A, Hara K, Kawai H, Yamamura Y, Mochizuki Y, Koshikawa T, Inada K. Endoscopic ultrasound-guided fine-needle aspiration biopsy for the diagnosis of gastrointestinal stromal tumors in the stomach. J Gastroenterol. 2004;39(8):747–53.

[62] Corless CL, Schroeder A, Griffith D, Town A, McGreevey L, Harrell P, Shiraga S, Bainbridge T, Morich J, Heinrich MC. PDGFRA mutations in gastrointestinal stromal tumors: frequency, spectrum and in vitro sensitivity to imatinib. J Clin Oncol. 2005,10;23(23):5357–64.

[63] Hunt GC, Rader AE, Faigel DO. A comparison of EUS features between CD-117 positive GI stromal tumors and CD-117 negative GI spindle cell tumors. Gastrointest Endosc. 2003;57(4):469–74.

[64] Fletcher CD, Berman JJ, Corless C, Gorstein F, Lasota J, Longley BJ, Miettinen M, O'Leary TJ, Remotti H, Rubin BP, Shmookler B, Sobin LH, Weiss SW. Diagnosis of gastrointestinal stromal tumors: a consensus approach. Hum Pathol. 2002;33(5):459–65.

[65] Seremetis MG, Lyons WS, deGuzman VC, Peabody JW Jr. Leiomyomata of the esophagus. An analysis of 838 cases. Cancer. 1976;38(5):2166–77.

[66] Lee LS, Singhal S, Brinster CJ, Marshall B, Kochman ML, Kaiser LR, Kucharczuk JC. Current management of esophageal leiomyoma. Am Coll Surg. 2004;198(1):136–46.

[67] Fernandez MJ, Davis RP, Nora PF. Gastrointestinal lipomas. Arch Surg. 1983;118(9):1081–3.

[68] Parmar JH, Lawrence R, Ridley NT. Submucous lipoma of the ileocaecal valve presenting as caecal volvulus. Int J Clin Pract. 2004;58(4):424–5.

[69] Watanabe F, Honda S, Kubota H, Higuchi R, Sugimoto K, Iwasaki H, Yoshino G, Kanamaru H, Hanai H, Yoshii S, Kaneko E. Preoperative diagnosis of ileal lipoma by endoscopic ultrasonography probe. J Clin Gastroenterol. 2000;31(3):245–7.

[70] Zhou PH, Yao LQ, Zhong YS, et al. Role of endoscopic miniprobe ultrasonography in diagnosis of submucosal tumor of large intestine. World J Gastroenterol. 2004,15;10(16):2444–6.

[71] Buscaglia JM, et al. Diagnostic yield and safety of jumbo biopsy forceps in patients with subepithelial lesions of the upper and lower GI tract. Gastrointest Endosc. 2012;75(6):1147–52.

[72] Thompson WM, Kende AI, Levy AD. Imaging characteristics of gastric lipomas in 16 adult and pediatric patients. AJR Am J Roentgenol. 2003 Oct;181(4):981–5.

[73] Garcia M, Buitrago E, Bejarano PA, Casillas J. Large esophageal liposarcoma: a case report and review of the literature. Arch Pathol Lab Med. 2004;128(8):922–5.

[74] Yoshizawa A, Ota H, Sakaguchi N, Kanai S, Nakayama J, Matsuzawa K, Tsuzuki S, Takada R, Miyazawa F, Kasahara H, Katsuyama T. Malignant granular cell tumor of the esophagus. Virchows Arch. 2004;444(3):304–6.

[75] Prematilleke IV, Piris J, Shah KA. Fine needle aspiration cytology of a granular cell tumour of the oesophagus. Cytopathology. 2004;15(2):120–1.

[76] De Ceglie A, Gatteschi B, Blanchi S, Scotto F, Pellecchia A, Conio M. Esophageal granular cell tumor treated by endoscopic mucosal resection. A case report and review of the literature. Dig Dis Sci. 2005;50(10):1875–9.

[77] Jovanovic I, Knezevic S, Micev M, Krstic M. EUS mini probes in diagnosis of cystic dystrophy of duodenal wall in heterotopic pancreas: a case report. World Gastroenterol. 2004,1;10(17):2609–12.

[78] Matsushita M, Hajiro K, Okazaki K, Takakuwa H. Gastric aberrant pancreas: EUS analysis in comparison with the histology. Gastrointest Endosc. 1999;49(4 Pt 1):493–7.

[79] Shalaby M, Kochman ML, Lichtenstein GR. Heterotopic pancreas presenting as dysphagia. Am J Gastroenterol. 2002;97(4):1046–9.

[80] Faigel DO, Gopal D, Weeks DA, Corless C. Cap-assisted endoscopic submucosal resection of a pancreatic rest. Gastrointest Endosc. 2001;54(6):782–4.

[81] Modlin IM, Lye KD, Kidd M. A 5-decade analysis of 13,715 carcinoid tumors. Cancer. 2003,15;97(4):934–59.

[82] Modlin IM, Lye KD, Kidd M. A 50-year analysis of 562 gastric carcinoids: small tumor or larger problem? Am J Gastroenterol. 2004;99(1):23–32.

[83] Soga J. Early-stage carcinoids of the gastrointestinal tract: an analysis of 1914 reported cases. Cancer. 2005,15;103(8):1587–95.

[84] Ichikawa J, Tanabe S, Koizumi W, Kida Y, Imaizumi H, Kida M, Saigenji K, Mitomi H. Endoscopic mucosal resection in the management of gastric carcinoid tumors. Endoscopy. 2003;35(3):203–6.

[85] Kwaan MR, Goldberg JE, Bleday R. Rectal carcinoid tumors: review of results after endoscopic and surgical therapy. Arch Surg. 2008;143(5):471–5.

[86] Kobayashi K, Katsumata T, Yoshizawa S, Sada M, Igarashi M, Saigenji K, Otani Y. Indications of endoscopic polypectomy for rectal carcinoid tumors and clinical usefulness of endoscopic ultrasonography. Dis Colon Rectum. 2005;48(2):285–91.

[87] Modlin IM, Kidd M, Latich I, Zikusoka MN, Shapiro MD. Current status of gastrointestinal carcinoids. Gastroenterology. 2005;128(6):1717–51.

[88] Ramage JK, et al. Guidelines for the management of gastroenteropancreatic neuroendocrine (including carcinoid) tumours. Gut. 2005;54(Suppl 4):1–16.

[89] Romero-Castro R, Pellicer-Bautista FJ, Jimenez-Saenz M, Marcos-Sanchez F, Caunedo-Alvarez A, Ortiz-Moyano C, Gomez-Parra M, Herrerias-Gutierrez JM. EUS-guided injection of cyanoacrylate in perforating feeding veins in gastric varices: results in 5 cases. Gastrointest Endosc. 2007;66(2):402–7.

[90] Levy MJ, Wong Kee Song LM, Kendrick ML, Misra S, Gostout CJ. EUS-guided coil embolization for refractory ectopic variceal bleeding (with videos). Gastrointest Endosc. 2008;67(3):572–4.

[91] Binmoeller KF, Weilert F, Shah JN, Kim J. EUS-guided transesophageal treatment of gastric fundal varices with combined coiling and cyanoacrylate glue injection (with videos). Gastrointest Endosc. 2011;74(5):1019–25.

[92] Ott DJ, Wolfman NT, Wu WC, Chen MY, White WL. Endoscopic ultrasonography of benign esophageal cyst simulating leiomyoma. J Clin Gastroenterol. 1992;15:85–7.

[93] Faigel DO, Burke A, Ginsberg GG, Stotland BR, Kadish SL, Kochman ML. The role of endoscopic ultrasound in the evaluation and management of foregut duplications. Gastrointest Endosc. 1997;45(1):99–103.

[94] Baek YH, Choi SR, Lee BE, Kim GH. Gastric glomus tumor: analysis of endosonographic characteristics and computed tomographic findings. Dig Endosc. 2013;25(1):80–3.

[95] Yan SL, Yeh YH, Chen CH, Yang CC, Kuo CL, Wu HS. Gastric glomus tumor: a hypervascular submucosal tumor on power Doppler endosonography. J Clin Ultrasound. 2007;35(3):164–8.

[96] Tang M, Hou J, Wu D, Han XY, Zeng MS, Yao XZ. Glomus tumor in the stomach: computed tomography and endoscopic ultrasound findings. World J Gastroenterol. 2013,28;19(8):1327–9.

[97] Matsushita M, Hajiro K, Okazaki K, Takakuwa H. Endoscopic features of gastric inflammatory fibroid polyps. Am J Gastroenterol. 1996;91(8):1595–8.

[98] Matsushita M, Hajiro K, Okazaki K, Takakuwa H. Gastric inflammatory fibroid polyps: endoscopic ultrasonographic analysis in comparison with the histology. Gastrointest Endosc. 1997;46(1):53–7.

[99] Brooks JJ, Enterline HT. Primary gastric lymphomas. A clinicopathologic study of 58 cases with long-term follow-up and literature review. Cancer. 1983,15;51(4):701–11.

[100] Bolondi L, Casanova P, Caletti GC, Grigioni W, Zani L, Barbara L. Primary gastric lymphoma versus gastric carcinoma: endoscopic US evaluation. Radiology. 1987;165(3):821–6.

[101] Kim EY. Diagnosis of subepithelial lesion: still "tissue is the issue". Clin Endosc. 2013;46(4):313–4.

[102] Lee CK, Chung IK, Lee SH, Lee SH, Lee TH, Park SH, Kim HS, Kim SJ, Cho HD. Endoscopic partial resection with the unroofing technique for reliable tissue diagnosis of upper GI subepithelial tumors originating from the muscularis propria on EUS (with video). Gastrointest Endosc. 2010;71(1):188–94.

[103] Pellisé Urquiza M, Fernández-Esparrach G, Solé M, Colomo L, Castells A, Llach J, Mata A, Bordas JM, Piqué JM, Ginès A. Endoscopic ultrasound-guided fine needle aspiration: predictive factors of accurate diagnosis and cost-minimization analysis of on-site pathologist. Gastroenterol Hepatol. 2007;30(6):319–24.

[104] Eckardt AJ, Adler A, Gomes EM, Jenssen C, Siebert C, Gottschalk U, Koch M, Röcken C, Rösch T. Endosonographic large-bore biopsy of gastric subepithelial tumors: a prospective multicenter study. Eur J Gastroenterol Hepatol. 2012;24(10):1135–44.

[105] Cağlar E, Hatemi I, Atasoy D, Sişman G, Sentürk H. Concordance of endoscopic ultrasonography-guided fine needle aspiration diagnosis with the final diagnosis in subepithelial lesions. Clin Endosc. 2013;46(4):379–83.

[106] Rong L, Kida M, Yamauchi H, Okuwaki K, Miyazawa S, Iwai T, Kikuchi H, Watanabe M, Imaizumi H, Koizumi W. Factors affecting the diagnostic accuracy of endoscopic ultrasonography-guided fine-needle aspiration (EUS-FNA) for upper gastrointestinal submucosal or extraluminal solid mass lesions. Dig Endosc. 2012;24(5):358–63.

[107] Suzuki T, Arai M, Matsumura T, Arai E, Hata S, Maruoka D, Tanaka T, Nakamoto S, Imazeki F, Yokosuka O. Factors associated with inadequate tissue yield in EUS-FNA for gastric SMT. ISRN Gastroenterol. 2011;2011:619128.

[108] Mekky MA, Yamao K, Sawaki A, Mizuno N, Hara K, Nafeh MA, Osman AM, Koshikawa T, Yatabe Y, Bhatia V. Diagnostic utility of EUS-guided FNA in patients with gastric submucosal tumors. Gastrointest Endosc. 2010;71(6):913–9.

[109] Hoda KM, Rodriguez SA, Faigel DO. EUS-guided sampling of suspected GI stromal tumors. Gastrointest Endosc. 2009;69(7):1218–23.

[110] Savides TJ, Donohue M, Hunt G, Al-Haddad M, Aslanian H, Ben-Menachem T, Chen VK, Coyle W, Deutsch J, DeWitt J, Dhawan M, Eckardt A, Eloubeidi M, Esker A, Gordon SR, Gress F, Ikenberry S, Joyce AM, Klapman J, Lo S, Maluf-Filho F, Nickl N, Singh V, Wills J, Behling C. EUS-guided FNA diagnostic yield of malignancy in solid pancreatic masses: a benchmark for quality performance measurement. Gastrointest Endosc. 2007;66(2):277–82.

[111] Moon JS. Role of endoscopic ultrasonography in guiding treatment plans for upper gastrointestinal subepithelial tumors. Clin Endosc. 2016;49(3):220–5.

[112] Săftoiu A, Vilmann P, Guldhammer Skov B, Georgescu CV. Endoscopic ultrasound (EUS)-guided Trucut biopsy adds significant information to EUS-guided fine-needle aspiration in selected patients: a prospective study. Scand J Gastroenterol. 2007;42(1):117–25.

[113] Kaffes AJ, Chen RY, Tam W, Norton I, Cho S, Devereaux B, Vaughan R. A prospective multicenter evaluation of a new side-port endoscopic ultrasound-fine-needle aspiration in solid upper gastrointestinal lesions. Dig Endosc. 2012;24(6):448–51.

[114] Lee HL. Advances in the management of upper gastrointestinal subepithelial tumor: pathologic diagnosis using endoscopy without endoscopic ultrasound-guided biopsy. Clin Endosc. 2016;49(3):216–9.

[115] Jeong ID, Jung SW, Bang SJ, Shin JW, Park NH, Kim DH. Endoscopic enucleation for gastric subepithelial tumors originating in the muscularis propria layer. Surg Endosc. 2011;25(2):468–74.

Section 2

Special Applications

Chapter 3

Endobronchial Ultrasound in Mediastinal Lymphadenopathy

Ilya V. Sivokozov, Olga. V. Lovacheva,
Irina. Y. Shabalina, Galina V. Evgushenko,
Tatyana A. Statsuk, Larisa N. Lepekha,
Yuri S. Berezovsky, Natalya N. Makaryants,
Larisa N. Chernousova and Elena E. Larionova

Additional information is available at the end of the chapter

http://dx.doi.org/10.5772/66079

Abstract

Currently, endobronchial ultrasound dramatically changed diagnostic approaches for mediastinal lesions, both benign and malignant. Still there is a lack of data regarding the optimal anaesthesia, route of intubation, needle type, and specific clinical situations concerning EBUS in real clinical practice. A short, but clinically oriented, description of EBUS-TBNA and EUS-b-FNA techniques for mediastinal lesions is provided.

Keywords: diagnostics, bronchoscopy, EBUS, EUS-b, sarcoidosis, tuberculosis, lung cancer, lymphoma

1. Introduction

From its first implementation [1] in clinical practice in 2003, convex endobronchial ultrasound-guided transbronchial needle aspiration (EBUS-TBNA) has rapidly evolved into one of the most hugely used diagnostic techniques in interventional pulmonology. Currently, all main companies in the field presented their systems for EBUS, with minor differences in modalities. Still there is a lack of data regarding the optimal anaesthesia, route of intubation, needle-type, and specific clinical situations, concerning EBUS in real clinical practice. Most recent CHEST panel recommendations, organized by AABIP/ACCP stated some unresolved issues with EBUS features, including anaesthesia type, needle choice, and others [2]. Interestingly, many recommendations were even ungraded by expert panel due to the absence of any studies covering exact questions. Thereafter, authors will share their own experience with EBUS and try to answer some of the issues in this area.

2. Indications and contraindications

Indications for EBUS/EUS-b are:

- Mediastinal adenopathy of unknown cause
- PET-positive LNs in mediastinum in patients with previous or current malignancy, irrespective of their size
- Suspected mediastinal cyst (normally evaluation only)
- Central lung cancer with failed conventional biopsies (peribronchial growth)
- Suspected tumour invasion into main vessels/mediastinal structures
- Transoesophageal LAG biopsy using bronchoscope

Contraindications:

- Severe thrombocytopenia (<25,000/mcl)
- Confirmed mediastinal cyst (if no other abnormalities seen on radiology)
- Non-correctable severe hypoxia
- Lack of personnel experience

3. Endobronchial ultrasound: equipment

Currently, all main companies in the field supply dedicated systems for EBUS, with minor differences in modalities. Main features of the equipment presented in **Table 1**.

Principally, there is no fundamental difference between the systems. Olympus and Fujinon have chosen a path to establish a separate, dedicated endoscopic ultrasound units, which can be mounted in an endoscopic tray, thus making procedure more convenient for personnel. Pentax systems have no dedicated endoscopic ultrasound centres, using instead a separate machines of high-level and expert class (e.g., Hitachi Noblus system). Apart from general EUS area, where ultrasound quality plays an essential role, EBUS situations do not impose such high requirements for quality of ultrasound image. Mobility, compact fashion and laconic interface are main features, which much more important for interventional pulmonologist, performing a procedure. Still, Olympus echobronchoscopes have a possibility to be connected with stand-alone machines (e.g., Aloka $\alpha7/\alpha10$), which can be a possible option for large endoscopic suites, where both EUS and EBUS are performed, giving a chance for a more optimal usage of these systems. Honestly, this variant is not currently popular.

There are several important things about echobronchoscopes. First of all, they all are very fragile and have to be used with great caution, and only for the purpose of EBUS, not for conventional procedures such as BAL, TBLB, etc. In frames of ease of use, Fuji scope is better to intubate and make an inspection of trachea and bronchial tree due to less oblique forward viewing (10° vs. 35° in Olympus and 45° in Pentax scopes) and high-definition image. One additional advantage of Fuji scope is that it allows to use conventional TBNA needles [3] during EBUS-TBNA procedure, when the other scopes have specific angulations of working channel, precluding insertion of conventional TBNA needle. The ultrasound field of view is a bit better in Fuji and especially Pentax comparing to Olympus, but in terms of biopsy procedure it does not make significant sense. From the other side, Olympus scope has a larger working channel diameter, which gives an opportunity to use 21G and even a 19G EBUS needles [4]. Pentax-based system (Hitachi Noblus) gives an access to latest generation of elastography and strain-ratio measurements, as also as additional features and options of ultrasound, given by a separate expert class machine, but the other side of the coin is less ease of use for such combination.

	Olympus	**Pentax**	**Fujinon**
Endoscope	**BF-UC180F**	**EB-1970UK**	**EB-530US**
Direction of view	35° forward oblique	45° forward oblique	10° forward oblique
Resolution	Standard, chip	Standard, chip	High Def, chip
Insertion tube o. d., (mm)	6.3	6.3	6.3
Channel diameter	2.2	2.0	2.0
Needle gauges	25-22-21-19	25-22	25-22
Main ultrasound systems	EU-ME1/ EU-ME2	Hitachi Noblus	Sonart SU-1
Scanning range, degrees	60	75	65
Colour and power Doppler	+/+	+	+
Tissue harmonic echo	–/+	+	–
Elastography	–/+	+	–
Contrast-enhanced US	–/+	–	–

Table 1. Main features of available EBUS systems.

In any case, all the scopes and systems provide the ability to perform intubation of trachea, inspection of bronchial tree, and needle biopsy of mediastinal and hilar structures for the vast majority of clinical situations.

4. Endosonography in mediastinal lesions: current status

For the last decade, EBUS implementation led to outstanding changes in management of respiratory patients, especially in lung cancer, sarcoidosis, tuberculosis and lymphoma.

Guidelines for diagnosis and treatment for lung cancer issued by ACCP [5] in May 2013 stated that in patients with suspected lung cancer with extensive mediastinal infiltration based on radiology and no evidence of metastatic disease, the diagnosis should be established including EBUS-TBNA or EUS-FNA, whatever technique is available and suitable for concrete patient. In the same guideline, in case of performing staging in patients with suspicion of N2-N3 disease, EBUS-TBNA, EUS-FNA or their combination are recommended over surgical staging as the best first step. Interestingly, that both these recommendations have a first-grade power, i.e., were confirmed by randomized clinical trials. In a more recent guideline, issued in June 2015 by ESGE/ERS/ESTS, dedicated to the role of EUS-EBUS in lung cancer diagnosis and staging [6], the main recommendation by experts was to use endosonography for staging in NSCLC patients over surgery as initial step (grade A), and if possible, to do that in combined fashion (EBUS-TBNA/EUS-FNA, or EBUS-TBNA/EUS-b-FNA) to achieve complete endoscopic staging (grade C).

Great number of publications were issued concerning the role of endosonography in sarcoidosis patients. Indeed, more than 80% of newly diagnosed sarcoidosis have mediastinal involvement by radiology. First paper, dedicated to EBUS-TBNA efficacy in sarcoidosis stage I, was published already in 2004 [7], showing the yield more than 90%. In frames of recent meta-analysis (more than 2000 cases of mediastinal adenopathy) published by Trisolini in 2015 [8], EBUS-TBNA was effective in 79% among sarcoidosis patients. Again, CHEST panel recommendations [2], issued in 2016, included suggestion to use EBUS-TBNA as first diagnostic modality for patients with suspicion of sarcoidosis. Surprisingly, international WASOG guidelines for diagnosis and treatment of sarcoidosis are extremely old and were issued in 1999, before new era of EBUS began, and still are not updated. Several countries in their national guidelines for sarcoidosis diagnostics and treatment already included EBUS-TBNA/EUS-FNA as a reliable technique in diagnostic workup in this cohort [8].

Tuberculosis, one of the most widespread infections on the global level, is also in the field of view for EBUS. Recent CHEST recommendations [2] have a suggestion to use EBUS-TBNA/EUS-FNA as suitable diagnostic modality for patients with suspicion of tuberculosis. Unfortunately, the data for endosonography in TB area are much weaker than in other diseases due high costs of this technique for low-income countries, which mostly suffer from high burden of tuberculosis.

Last, but not the least, lymphomas became a point if interest for endosonography in a last couple of years. Until recently, main option for such cohort of patients in primary diagnostics was surgical biopsy, due to need in a large amount of tissue with true biopsy specimen. When in 2014 EBUS tru-cut histology needles became available, situation began to change [9].

To improve the diagnostic yield, new imaging modalities enter now into EBUS area, arising from gastrointestinal endosonography. Among them—elastography—technique, which can

http://dx.doi.org/10.5772/66079

give as a non-invasive assessment of lesion stiffness and perform targeted biopsy; tissue harmonic echo, which diminishes artefacts from rapid motion and increases spatial resolution; and different contrast enhancement modes, allowing operator to assess vascularization patterns in mediastinal nodes or lesions to better characterize the origin of disease and perform precise interventions.

Besides that, a trend to change the focus from EBUS-guided biopsies to EBUS-guided interventions is clearly visible. In other words, now, we can diagnose the diseases of mediastinum effectively, and move on to the next step—to use this technique in treatment of patients. Some of these promising new goals—chemotherapy agent injections in locally advanced lung cancer, mediastinal cysts drainage, transvascular interventions—are discussed thereafter in this chapter.

5. Image modalities for EBUS/EUS-b

5.1. B-mode: grayscale

Grayscale mode, a basic mode for assessment of mediastinal structures, mainly lymphatic nodes (LN) during EBUS, can give a number of data for operator. LN size, echogenicity, shape, margins, central hilar structure, necrosis sign, invasion into main vessels of heart chambers can be estimated. Usually, main question for bronchologist, performing an EBUS investigation, is to distinguish benign and malignant adenopathy, because it has crucial impact on patient management. According to Fujiwara [10], who proposed a standard classification of EBUS image, features, typical for malignancy, are as follows: short axis size >10 mm, round shape, distinct margin, heterogeneous structure, hypoechoic, the absence of central hilar structure, and necrosis sign. If more than 4 of these criteria were met, calculated malignancy probability reached 96% (see **Figure 1**). Common features for benign lesions are—blurry margin, homogeneous structure, hyperechoic, the presence of central hilum, triangular or septate shape (see **Figure 2**).

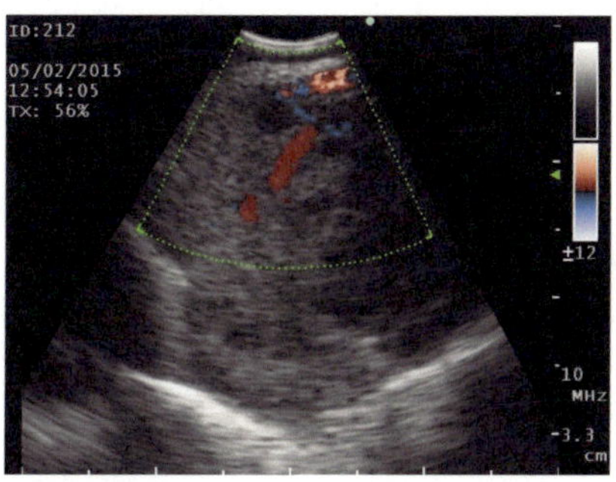

Figure 1. Malignant LN in mediastinal recurrence of renal cell carcinoma. Note hypoechoic character, heterogeneous structure, the presence of BA-flow (discussed afterwards). The presence of multiple necrosis signs in upper part of lesion is typical in patients after chemotherapy.

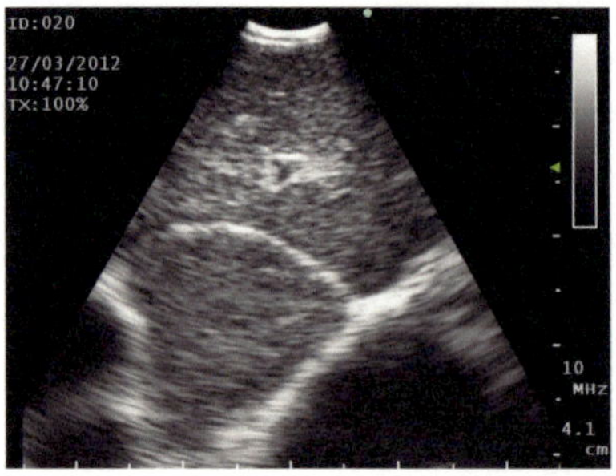

Figure 2. Benign LN in acute sarcoidosis. Note hyperechoic character, blurry margins, triangular shape, septated.

Of course, grayscale image cannot replace a biopsy, which is the gold standard for mediastinal lesions of any cause. Using B-mode, operator can choose, which of the lesions looks more suspicious for malignancy, or even choose an exact zone inside the node for biopsy.

5.2. Power and colour-flow Doppler

Doppler detects movement of fluid in the area of scanning. In theory, neovascularization in malignant LN can be traced by Doppler, and therefore, this technique can help to distinguish malignant lesion from benign. In 2012, Nakajima [11] proposed scoring system for blood flow in LN, from Grade 0 (no or small flow) through Grade 1 (few main vessels from hilum toward the centre), Grade 2 (few punctiforms or rod-shaped flow signals or a few small vessels found as a long strip of a curve) until Grade III (rich flow, more than four vessels found with different diameters or twist- or helical -low signal). The blood flow from the bronchial artery (BA) toward the LN was also recorded using Colour Doppler imaging as a sign for BA inflow. It was shown that Grades 0–1 were specific for benign lesion, whereas higher grades and especially BA sign—for malignancy with a tital accuracy around 80%. It needs to be emphasized, that only biopsy can confirm or exclude malignant or benign disease, and this is perfectly illustrated (see **Figures 3**, **4**).

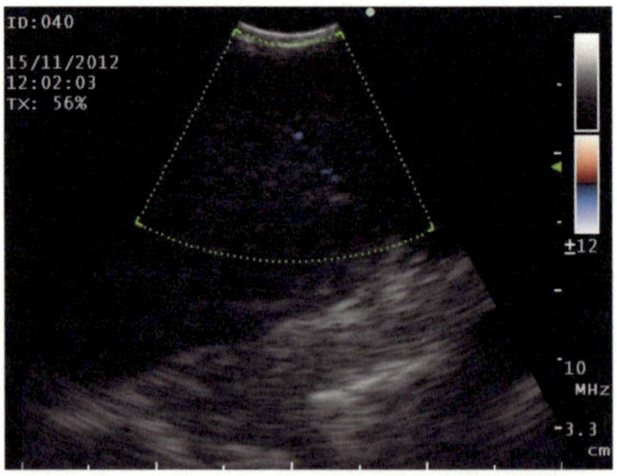

Figure 3. Large subcarinal LN in patient with metastatic adenocarcinoma. According to the Doppler flow (Grade 0–1 spot vessel), this LN can be falsely assessed as benign.

http://dx.doi.org/10.5772/66079

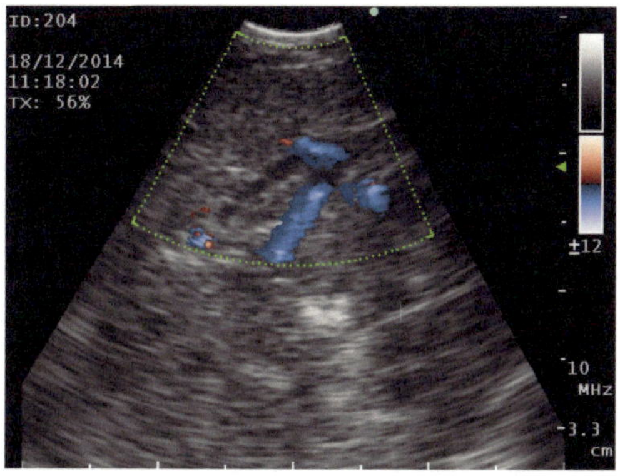

Figure 4. Large subcarinal LN, protruding to station 8 in patient with chronic sarcoidosis. According to the Doppler flow (Grade 3—number of large twisted vessels), this LN can be falsely assessed as malignant.

Use of Doppler during EBUS is irreplaceable when a biopsy is planned. This technique helps to plan a biopsy path, avoiding vessels inside LN, large vascular structures, heart chambers, thus providing a safe intervention. It should be noted that Colour Flow mode is less sensitive than power flow, so in difficult cases, when sludge is suspected, Power Doppler is more suitable option. Stand-alone ultrasound machines can reach even higher sensitivity, using special modes of vascular flow detection (e.g., Hitachi Noblus, see **Figure 5**).

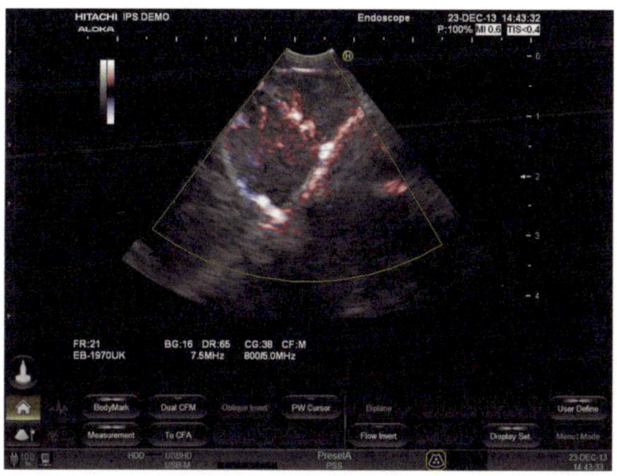

Figure 5. Subcarinal LN in patient with chronic sarcoidosis and concomitant pulmonary hypertension. eFlow regimen depicts vascular structures in septa between LN agglomeration, not detected in Colour Flow mode.

5.3. Elastography

One of the new modalities, which became available today for EBUS is elastography. This is an imaging procedure that can assess the biomechanical characteristics of different tissues and their deformation under compression [12]. Simplifying, elastography can measure stiffness of scanning area, where malignant tissue has lower elasticity and higher stiffness than benign. Currently, both Olympus and Pentax provided such a mode for EBUS. Independently of producer, a colour histogram reflecting stiffness of scanning area is superimposed on a grayscale image, where more blue colour means less elastic areas, and more green colour depicts more elastic areas. In other words—"blue is bad, green is good".

Two main logical applications for this technique are assessment of mediastinal LNs for probable malignancy during staging of NCLC, and performing a targeted EBUS-TBNA for a precise part of LN or group of them.

As elastography makes only first steps in respiratory world, the evidence of usefulness for this technique is still scarce. First publication for EBUS elastography was issued in 2013 [13] stated that this technique is feasible and can be performed in bronchial tree. In 2014, Izumo et al. [14] proposed classification of strain features of LNs based on the predominant colour at elastography investigation—predominantly blue, non-blue, or mixed, showing accuracy rate in malignancy detection more than 97%. The same year, in another study [15], feasibility of method in EBUS was confirmed, and impact of access (EBUS or EUS-b) on elastography results was depicted, showing probability to overestimate stiffness of the same lymphatic node using EBUS comparing to EUS-b approach. Rozman et al. [16] used a strain ratio—stiffness of targeted area divided by stiffness of reference area and came to conclusion that cut-off of ratio 8 and more predicts malignancy with positive predictive value of 81% and negative predictive value of 91%, which is the best efficacy than any other image modality for EBUS available nowadays.

Elastography can be used not only for mediastinal lesions assessment (see **Figure 6**). It can be utilized also for pulmonary masses, adjacent to bronchial tree or oesophagus (see **Figure 7**).

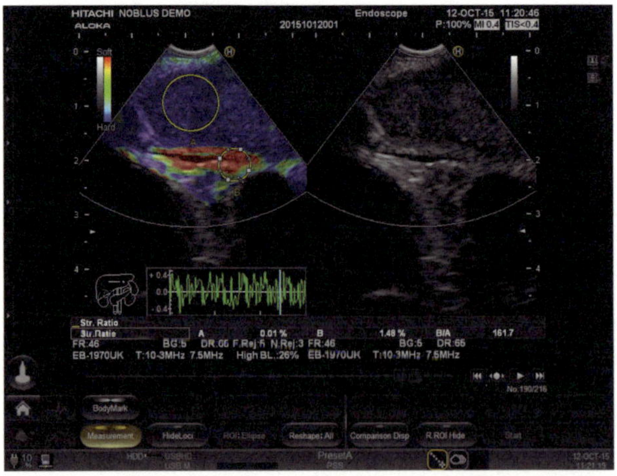

Figure 6. Huge subcarinal LN in patient with metastatic adenocarcinoma. Note the total blue colour on histogram, and two markers for strain ratio measurement, which far exceeded 120, suggesting malignant character of LN.

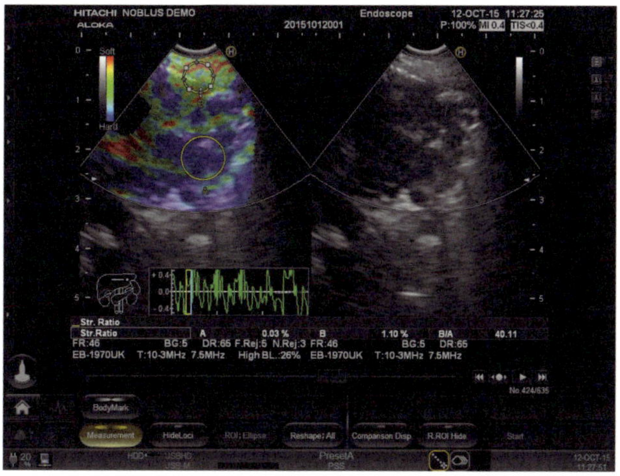

Figure 7. The same patient, lung mass is visible in right S6 adjacent to oesophagus, near the subcarinal LN. Note numerous echo artefacts on the mass border with aerated lung. Predominantly, blue-coloured area, SR exceeds 40. Metastatic adenocarcinoma.

5.4. Tissue harmonic echo (THE) and contrast-enhancement in EBUS

Several current systems for EBUS optionally can use both THE and contrast enhancement modes for endobronchial approach. Tissue harmonic echo is used for many years in digestive endosonography, namely for pancreatic lesions and hepatobiliary disorders [17]. Using a harmonic reflection instead of fundamental image can increase the signal ratio and thus give an opportunity to visualize structures more clear. Possible technique applications in mediastinum enclose better visualization of difficult-to-reach structures with low echogenicity, better assessment of tumour invasion in adjacent structures, etc.

The blood flow in small vessels and the parenchymal microvasculature of the target lesion can be observed non-invasively by contrast-enhanced EUS (CE-EUS). Through a hemodynamic analysis, CE-EUS permits the diagnosis of various gastrointestinal diseases and differential diagnoses between benign and malignant tumours [18]. It was shown that in mediastinal LNs CE-EUS can detect a filling defect, which is a typical sign of malignant lymphadenopathy, with a sensitivity of 100% and a specificity of 84% [19]. Thus, this indicates possibility for the application of this method in the differential diagnosis of mediastinal lymphadenopathy.

6. Endobronchial ultrasound-guided biopsies of mediastinum

6.1. Instruments

There is a long list of available biopsy needles for EBUS on the market. Basically, all the needles can be divided in two groups—cytology and dedicated histology needles. Comparison of some needle features is presented in **Table 2**.

	Length (mm)	Compatibility	Type
Olympus			
Vizishot 22G	40	Olympus	Cytology
Vizishot 21G	40	Olympus	Cytology
Vizishot 19G	40	Olympus	Histology
Cook Medical			
Echotip Ultra 22G	50	All	Cytology
Echotip ProCore 25G	50	All	Histology
Echotip ProCore 22G	50	All	Histology
Boston Scientific			
Expect Pulmonary 25G	60	Olympus	Cytology
Expect Pulmonary 22G	60	Olympus	Cytology
MediGlobe			
SonoTip EBUS Pro	40	All	Cytology
SonoTip EBUS Pro Flex	40	All	Cytology

Table 2. Main features of available EBUS needles.

There are little data available regarding comparative efficacy of different EBUS needles both in frames of cytology/histology quality or diagnostic yield. Regarding 21 and 22G needles, still there is only one randomized trial by Oki [20], where no difference was seen in terms of adequacy or diagnostic yield. The same results were achieved by several other studies [21–23]. In other study by Izumo [24], compared Olympus and MediGlobe EBUS 22G needles, the latter showed better efficacy in terms of histology and total yield (74 vs. 61%). Notably, this study was not randomized and used Olympus needle as a historical control group. In a recent pre-published study by Xing et al. [25], EBUS ProCore needle was compared to ordinary cytology EBUS-TBNA needle (exact gauge was not stated), with respective efficacy of 94 and 89%. Authors did not state, what kind of patients they studied, and the data are resembling those for patients with benign or typical malignancy diseases, whereas ProCore needle was mostly expected to be used in difficult situations like lymphoma. There was a small randomized comparative study of Olympus and Cook 22G cytology EBUS needles [26], where in terms of cytology both needles show equal efficacy, but total diagnostic yield and yield by histology favoured Cook needle.

Finally, taking into account, some of the studies mentioned above, CHEST panel of experts [2] recommended use any type of needle, either 21 or 22G as an acceptable option (Grade 1C). From personal experience, authors would recommend to use any needle in case of benign disease or NSCLC for typical LN stations, and histology EBUS needles (19G Olympus or 22–25G ProCoreCook) in case of suspected lymphoma, or if definitive pathology diagnosis should be established. Smaller needle size (22–25G) can be an advantage in specific situations—like lesions in stations 2R/L, 4L, 11-12R/L, transvascular interventions.

6.2. Balloon: use or not?

All EBUS scopes have possibility to use a special balloon over their distal ultrasound tip, filled with saline for better contact of the probe with bronchial wall in challenging situations. Unfortunately, still there are no studies available to assess the real sense of this additional and disposable equipment. Balloons are widely accepted in routine practice in Northern America, and CHEST recommendations [2] on EBUS suggest their usage for paratracheal lesions and hilar stations. In Europe and Japan, balloon usage is much less popular, at least partially due to possibility to use transoesophageal approach for 7 and 4L stations via EUS-b procedures.

From personal experience, authors recommend balloon usage for the beginners in EBUS. With increased experience usage of balloon can be avoided in a vast majority of clinical situations.

6.3. Anaesthesia and intubation way

Endobronchial ultrasound can be performed in different anaesthesia settings—conscious sedation, general anaesthesia, or even local anaesthesia. Interestingly, that firstly EBUS-TBNA was performed mostly under local anaesthesia, and only in a couple of years after sedation was generally accepted [27]. Currently, moderate or deep sedation is recommended as the main anaesthesia way for EBUS by recent guidelines [2], but evidence level for that is not so good (Grade 2C). Studies dedicated to comparison of deep versus moderate sedation showed conflicting results, precluding clear algorithm of anaesthesia in EBUS procedure.

From personal experience, authors recommend to use all mentioned above ways of anaesthesia, but starting from exact situation. Thus, for example, local anaesthesia is still an option when a diagnostic procedure with single biopsy is planned, especially in case of EUS-b approach for enlarged LN in positions 7 and 4L. If an EBUS approach is planned, local anaesthesia still can be used, especially with transcricoid injection of 2% lidocaine. This type of anaesthesia provides adequate control over laryngeal and cough reflex, giving an opportunity to perform procedure with extremely high patient compliance for 15–20 min.

Sedation, deep or conscious, can be recommended in situations where procedure duration exceeds 15 min, LAG biopsy with EBUS scope is indicated, multiple biopsies planned (staging), or technical issues during puncture are foreseen.

General anaesthesia can be recommended in several situations—during EBUS implementation in clinic, when an operator is not very experienced, or if other anaesthesia types are not safe for patient, or in case of extremely long procedure (i.e., full staging of all assessable LN stations).

There are several ways of intubation with EBUS bronchoscope. It can be inserted alone via transoral or transnasal approach or can be inserted via artificial airways—laryngeal mask, intubation tube, or rigid scope. Again, data from studies referred for this question are extremely scarce and cannot give any definitive suggestion which variant of intubation is better. Based on personal experience, authors recommend further indications: use transoral approach during EBUS under local anaesthesia only. If it is sometimes needed to intubate through the nasal cavity, remember that this is slightly more difficult due to larger endoscope diameter, rigid distal part, and oblique optics. Choosing between laryngeal mask and intubation tube, we recommend fist option, because intubation tube limits as mobility of endoscope inside bronchial tree, as a visibility of some LN stations, like 2L/R, 4L/R, 3p. besides that, a cuff of a tube can damage the sheath of a scope, especially during staging procedures. Also, multiple scope passes in and out of intubation tube can lead to a more rapid degradation of this fragile equipment. The last option for EBUS intubation—through a rigid scope. This variant has only advantage over others—due to straight way of the barrel, EBUS scope have a less chance to be damaged during biopsy, and lower degradation rate due to less active bending. All the rest is not in favour of this method—so, scope can be damaged by retraction, angulation, and rotation during scanning and puncture, especially for 4L position. Besides that, upper paratracheal LN groups, as 3p group is not achievable using this approach.

Last, but not the least, it needs to be mentioned that echobronchoscope can be inserted not only in trachea, but also into oesophagus, thus obtaining an opportunity to reach 7 and especially 4L positions much more easy than through trachea, and widens assessable biopsy area to station 8, 9 and even LAG. This is called an EUS-b approach, and according to latest European guidelines [6], this method is encouraged to be used by respiratory care professionals for complete endoscopic staging in NSCLC. In North America, unfortunately, bronchologists are under severe pressure of regulations, and this limits spread of this very simple and convenient, both for doctor and patient, procedure.

6.4. Biopsy technique: movement, suction, stylet and more

Analyzing biopsy step by step, a huge decision tree for operator can be seen. Hereafter, each step of procedure will be discussed with relevant comments.

Stylet. Each needle has a stylet, which blocks an inner lumen to avoid contamination of specimen, and additionally, protects working channel from damage as needle passes through the scope. There are two options—to use stylet or not. Currently, there is no dedicated publications for this question regarding EBUS. But, taking into account recent meta-analysis of this issue for EUS-FNA [28] with more than 5000 cases included, it can be suggested that stylet possibly should not be used always during EBUS or EUS-b biopsies. From personal experience, authors recommend not to reinsert the stylet after first pass was performed, as it saves time of procedure, except needles where it is noted by manufacturer (MediGlobe) or needles with tru-cut design (ProCore), where stylet should be reinserted all the times to avoid working channel damage.

Suction. There are several options regarding suction: use, not use, apply "capillary" or "wet" approach. Capillary technique, or "slow-pull", means slow withdraw of stylet from needle, thus creating a residual vacuum inside needle to aspirate specimen. "Wet" approach means filling of needle lumen with saline, thus increasing the power of conventional suction syringe. Again, both recent guidelines for EBUS [2, 29] stated equal possibility to use suction or not.

http://dx.doi.org/10.5772/66079

Personally, authors recommend during first pass apply half-syringe suction; if specimen is too bloody, proceed without suction or "capillary" technique, if specimen is poor, apply full suction with further option to use "wet" approach. Additionally, if a high vascular pattern is seen by ultrasound imaging, it is recommended to start biopsy without suction or use "capillary" way.

Biopsy movements. Needle motions can be different by speed, force, and number. There are no studies comparing these approaches in terms of biopsy quality and efficacy. Hereafter, authors' opinion on their usage can be found.

- *RiSo—Rapid In, Slow Out*. Means rapid, forceful needle penetration into target, and slow return back. Fills up the needle-like a pipe. Recommended for LNs with low to intermediate vascular flow, and for ProCore needles.
- *SiSo—Slow In, Slow Out*. Means gentle, slow movement back and forth with low frequency. Suitable for highly vascularized lesions.
- *RiRo—Rapid In, Rapid Out*. Means rapid, forceful movements in both directions with high frequency. Option for rigid and stone-like lesions (e.g., lymphoma).
- *SiRo—Slow In, Rapid Out*. Means slow and gentle movement forward with more rapid way back. Rare option can be applied using 25G EUS ProCore needles through the bronchoscope, where cutting edge looks back; also can be used if a large vessel in LN cannot be avoided, providing careful entrance into the lesion.

Fanning. To cover larger amount of tissue inside the lesion, needle can change its path for each new movement, using control lever of the scope. This is called fanning, as it resembles the movements of a fan. Recommended for usage in most of situations as helps to sample more target areas.

Number of needle movements inside the LN. No data available. Authors recommend 15–20 needle agitations during single pass.

Number of passes. According to recent guidelines [2, 29], not <3 consecutive passes should be performed for each LN in case of NSCLC staging procedure. No data available regarding benign diseases. Authors recommend for benign diseases to perform at least 2 passes from each target LN, and in case of core retrieval avoid third pass.

6.5. Preparation of smears, cellblocks and culture

Smears should be prepared immediately after the material was expelled, or flushed from the needle. At first, specimen has to be macroscopically assessed (volume, colour, character, thickness, the presence of artificial fills). This can give an operator a chance to use the specimen more effectively. Any additional inclusions—looking like flocs, crumbs, firm strings, or nubbles of pus, should be evaluated. Any specimen, is it abundant or poor, bloody or not, can be used for cytology analysis (**Figure 8**).

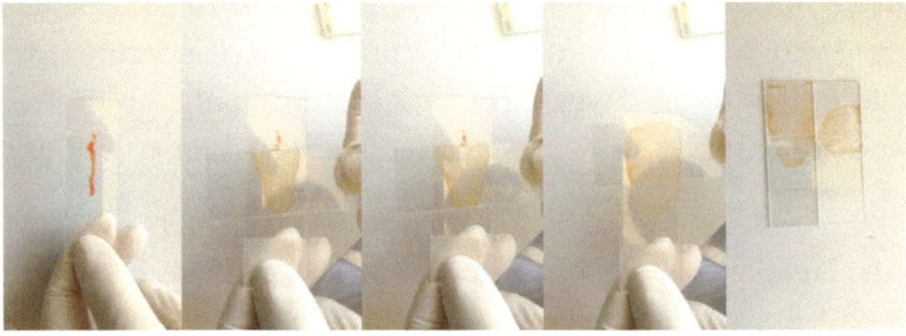

Figure 8. Steps of proper smear preparation from typical EBUS-TBNA specimen (from left to right).

In case of excessive blood contamination, smears should be prepared immediately to avoid clots formation, which will preclude the procedure. If specimen is liquid, it can be processed just like a blood smear (see **Figure 9**). If retrieved specimen is more solid, additionally smears can be achieved just rolling the solid component on the slide with a needle tip (see **Figure 10**). In other way, if retrieved specimen is too sticky, operator can put another slide from above and gently pressing, achieve the so-called touch smear (see **Figure 11**). All the movements and pressure should be applied to specimen with gentle force to avoid cells damage. In case of liquid, high-volume (>1 ml) specimen, it can be processed with centrifugation and consequent smears from precipitate. Notably, even low-volume specimens (<1 ml) can be processed using a cyto-spin.

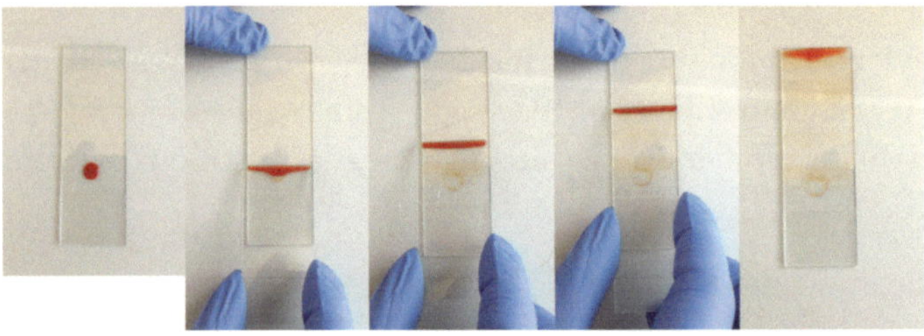

Figure 9. Steps of smear preparation from bloody specimen. Note clearly seen circle-shaped artefact due to clot formation, emphasizing need in immediate processing of such specimen.

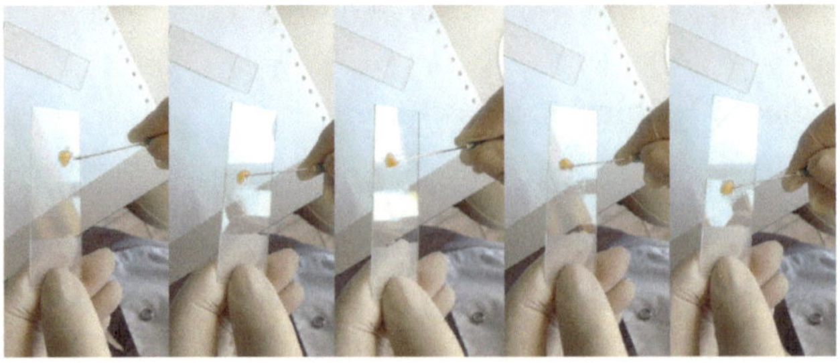

Figure 10. Steps of smear preparation from solid EBUS-TBNA specimen by rolling it by needle tip.

http://dx.doi.org/10.5772/66079

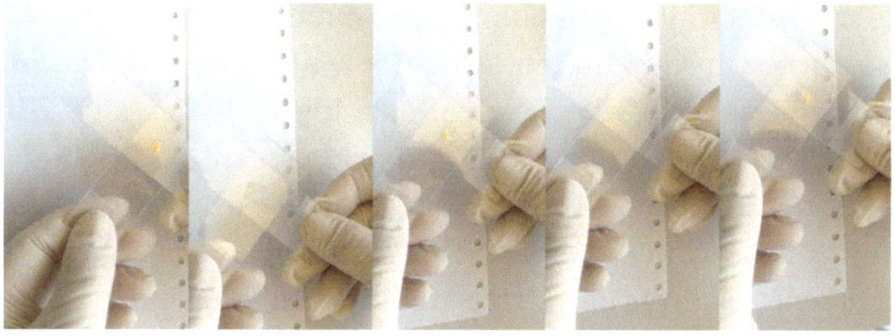

Figure 11. Steps of smear preparation from solid specimen by "touch smear" technique. Note that slides are moving after each touch, achieving sequential touch smears.

After air-dry, smears are stained for cytological examination. There are several staining methods available, and it depends on the local clinical practice of cytopathology or cytology laboratory.

If obtained specimen contains cores, it can be processed by two ways. Core tissue should be taken with care by tweezers or medical needle tip and placed directly to buffered 10% formalin solution; or core can be temporarily transferred to the filter paper to give blood to sink in paper, living core tissue free, and shortly after transfer the core into formalin. Most of this material is not a pure histology specimen, rather the so-called "cell block", which is though suitable for processing in pathology laboratory with all possible staining.

In case of suspected tuberculosis of other infection, both PCR and culture tests should be performed. This can be carried out by performing additional EBUS-TBNA pass with consequent flushing or expelling the specimen into transport medium; also, after last pass processing, EBUS needle can be flushed with saline into transport medium. No formal recommendations exist for microbiological investigation. Authors recommend flush EBUS needle with 10–15 ml of saline to achieve enough material volume for both tests for TB.

7. EBUS-guided interventions

7.1. Mediastinal cysts drainage

For a long time, mediastinal cyst was a contraindication for EBUS-TBNA or EUS-FNA procedures, due to high risk of consequent infection and surgical interventions. Till now, the most common pathway for such a patient can be formulated as "no symptoms—no treatment, any symptoms—surgery". Cystic lesions present some sort of a challenge for surgeon, that is why most of the cysts are not operated until they become symptomatic.

In 2007, Nakajima [30] published a fist case of EBUS procedure performed to for diagnostic, but for curative intent in a patient with severe central airway stenosis due to mediastinal cyst, without any complication or cyst recurrence. Three years later, even infected mediastinal cyst was successfully treated by EBUS-TBNA [31]. Importantly, in this case, puncture allowed not only to evacuate debris, but also perform culture analysis and thus prescribe appropriate antibiotics. This case also showed possibility for numerous punctures of the same lesion, providing stepwise approach to treatment. In 2015, Maturu et al. [32] performed first meta-analysis of mediastinal cysts drainage publications, found 16 cases of EBUS-TBNA for this indication. The overall complication rate after cyst drainage under EBUS-guidance was 18.7% (3 cases of complications, including cyst infection and pericarditis, cyst rupture and pneumonia, and mediastinitis), according to authors, this rate is comparable with surgical morbidity. Data regarding recurrence chances are scarce and non-reliable.

In conclusion, EBUS-TBNA for mediastinal cyst drainage is a possible option for at least some of cases. This can be a suitable alternative for surgery, or a salvation therapy for non-surgical candidates. Further studies needed to establish real value of such technique.

7.2. Chemotherapy agent injections in lung cancer

EBUS-TBNA became a standard of care in lung cancer patients. Possibility to precisely detect position of malignant LN and perform a biopsy in real-time fashion led to hypothesis of possible usage of endobronchial ultrasound for therapy agent injection in affected LN.

In 2013, first publication was performed regarding this issue by Brachmann group [33]. They used EBUS-TBNA with curative intent (named by authors TBND—transbronchial needle dosage) for regional metastatic LNs in six patients with stage IIIa-IV NSCLC, with six passes of cisplatin injections inside the lesion to cover the whole LN volume. Safety and possible efficacy of EBUS-TBND was shown. Two years later, in the end of 2015, Mehta et al. [34] reported first experience of lung cancer mediastinal and hilar recurrence EBUS-TBNI (I-injection) treatment with cisplatin in 36 patients. Response rate reached 69%, with significantly higher both overall and progression-free survival among responders.

In this way, EBUS-guided injection of chemotherapy is possible new paradigm for patient with locally advanced and recurrent NSCLC, not suitable for surgical resection.

8. Complications

From the beginning of EBUS implementation, it was stated that procedure is very safe, probably transferring experience available for conventional TBNA. Early sporadic case reports were interchanged with meta-analyses, when number of procedures has grown dramatically. According to the recent paper of Annema group [35], included more than 16,000 cases of EBUS/EUS performed for mediastinal lesions, severe adverse event rate was estimated as 0.05% for EBUS-TBNA, and minor adverse events rate was 0.22%, or around 1 in every 500 procedures. Authors came to conclusions that rate of minor adverse events is severely underestimated. Most of described in the literature EBUS-TBNA complications include infections of mediastinum (mediastinitis, abscess, pericarditis), pneumothorax, severe haemorrhage, and hypoxemia during and after procedure. It should be noted that most of infectious complications were caused by mediastinal cystic lesions, punctured by mistake without further drainage.

http://dx.doi.org/10.5772/66079

Among sarcoidosis patients, according to Agarwal et al. [36], minor adverse events were noted in 0.9% of cases. In elderly patients with lung cancer (>70-year old), complication rate was much higher and reached 5.8% [37]. Interestingly, in case of tuberculosis, rate of minor complications was calculated as 2.33% [38], and for severe as 0.12% [39] by two separate meta-analyses.

In conclusion, complications of EBUS-TBNA are rare, but not as rare as one might think. Each patient should be carefully observed after procedure to provide appropriate care for any consequent health problems.

9. Efficacy of EBUS-guided biopsies in specific diseases: clinical cases

9.1. Sarcoidosis and sarcoid-like reactions

Sarcoidosis stages I and II is one of the most common indications for EBUS-TBNA. According to the recent guidelines [2], EBUS-TBNA is recommended for diagnosis in patients with suspected sarcoidosis with mediastinal and/or hilar adenopathy. Efficacy of endosonography in diagnosing sarcoidosis varies—from 90% in highly selected population in 2004 [7], till 79% in routine practice in 2015 [40]. Mostly LN groups 7 and 4R are biopsied using EBUS approach, and station 7 and 4L—using EUS-b approach. In countries with high burden of TB, authors strongly recommend perform culture and PCR tests to avoid misinterpretation of granulomas in specimens.

Sarcoid-like reactions can accompany different malignancies, including NSCLC and lymphoma, sometimes mimic recurrence of main disease. They are seen in 4.4% of all solid tumours, and in almost 14% of patients with Hodgkin's lymphoma. In case of suspicion for such reaction, EBUS-TBNA can be performed to exclude or confirm malignancy.

Sometimes this reaction can coexist with tumour in the same lymphatic node (see **Figure 12**).

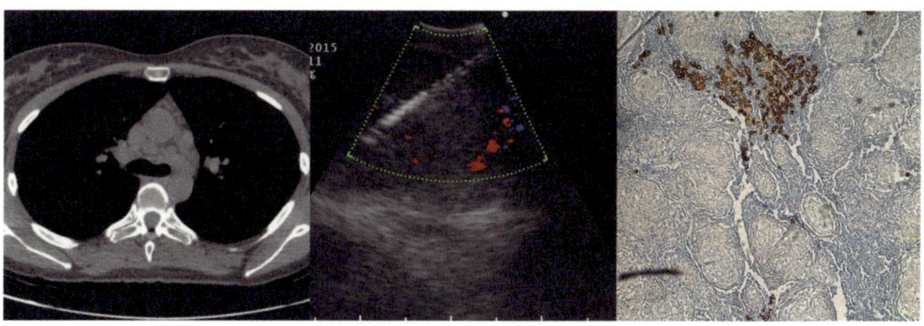

Figure 12. Patient with asymptomatic mediastinal adenopathy on chest CT (left), for suspected sarcoidosis EBUS-TBNA of LN 4R was performed using 21G Vizishot needle (middle, note the needle echo inside LN), pathology IHC with DAB staining for pancytokeratin revealing brown malignant cells, surrounded by multiple sarcoid granulomas (right). Metastatic adenocarcinoma coexisted with sarcoid-like reaction.

9.2. Primary and metastatic cancers

Both diagnosis and staging of lung cancer changed dramatically due to EBUS-TBNA implementation. Current guidelines for NSCLC diagnostics and staging [5, 6] recommend usage of endosonography for both mentioned indications as a first step, over a traditional surgical approach. The overall sensitivity and negative predictive value of EBUS-TBNA staging in NSCLC reaches 89 and 91%, respectively. New imaging modalities give a chance to further improve performance of lung cancer staging (see **Figure 13**).

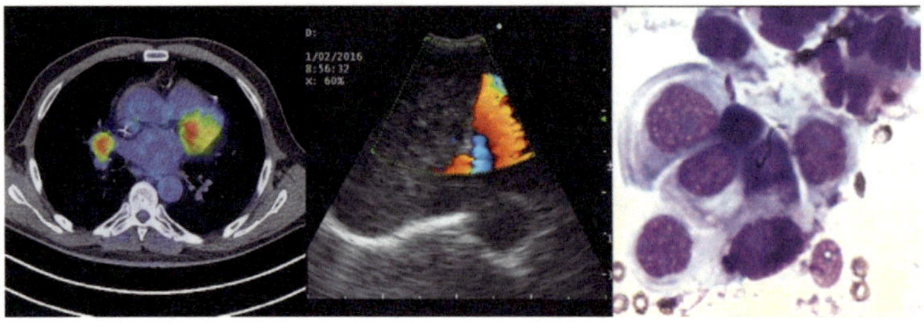

Figure 13. Patient with renal cell carcinoma in anamnesis with PET-positive R12 LN (left), for suspected cancer recurrence EBUS-TVNA (transvacular) was performed using 22G ProFlex needle (middle, note that brunch of RPV flows closely to the lesion), cytology (Giemza staining) showed malignant cells (right). Metastatic RCC recurrence.

9.3. Tuberculosis

Tuberculosis is not a popular indication for EBUS because of two main reasons. In countries where EBUS is available, tuberculosis has low prevalence, and reversely—in countries with high TB burden EBUS is too costly procedure to be routinely used for this indication. Nevertheless, several recent meta-analyses [38, 39] showed its sensitivity in patients with TB of 80%. Based on personal experience, authors recommend perform culture, PCR test and Ziel-Nielsen staining in all cases of suspected TB infection, because each investigation modality has an additive effect for final diagnostic yield (see **Figure 14**).

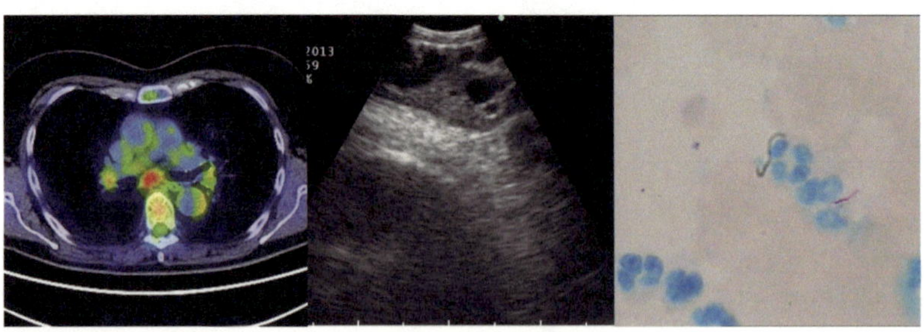

Figure 14. Patient with fever of unknown cause with Hodgkin's lymphoma anamnesis, with PET-positive 7 LN (left), for suspected lymphoma recurrence underwent EBUS-TBNA using 22G ProCore needle (middle, note multiple hypoechoic lesions—necrosis zones), cytology (Ziel-Nielsen staining) showed AFB, both PCR and Bactec tests were positive (right). Mediastinal LN tuberculosis.

9.4. Lymphoma

For decades, diagnosis of lymphoma was mostly surgical. Nowadays, situation began to change dramatically, and EBUS-TBNA becomes a suitable option for this indication [2]. Diagnosis of this disease is a real challenge both for clinician, bronchologist, and cytopathologist. According to the latest data [41], overall sensitivity of EBUS-TBNA in mediastinal lymphomas varies greatly from 38 to 91%, with further surgical confirmation needed in 13–43% of patients. Even in the worst scenario, EBUS-TBNA can possibly lower the need in surgical diagnosis of lymphoma more than by half. As new biopsy instruments and image modalities become available, efficacy of EBUS-TBNA for this indication will apparently increase (see **Figure 15**).

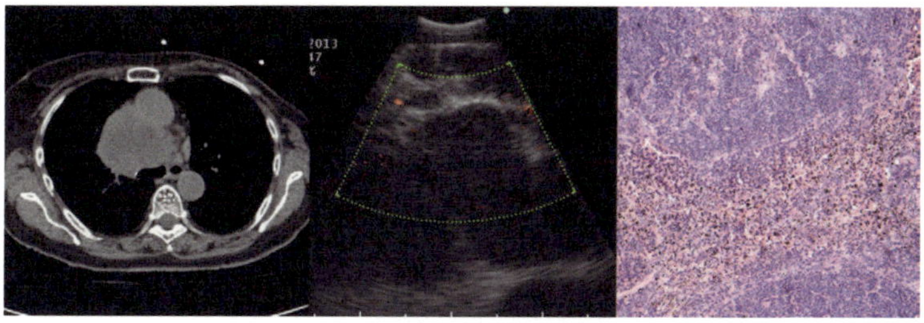

Figure 15. Patient with anterior mediastinal of unknown origin (left), for suspected lymphoma underwent EBUS-TBNA using 22G ProCore needle (middle, note huge hypoechoic mass without blood flow by power Doppler), pathology with HE staining showed widened mantle zone with prominent lymphoid tissue, consequent IHC confirmed Hodgkin's disease (right).

10. Conclusion

Endobronchial ultrasound is a powerful and effective instrument to diagnose mediastinal adenopathies. This technology already changed patient management strategies in sarcoidosis and lung cancer and starts to change situation in tuberculosis and lymphoma. Further developments in imaging modalities and biopsy equipment will give a chance to go beyond current indications of EBUS, provide a new step from diagnosis to treatment of both malignant and benign diseases.

Author details

Ilya V. Sivokozov*, Olga. V. Lovacheva, Irina. Y. Shabalina, Galina V. Evgushenko, Tatyana A. Statsuk, Larisa N. Lepekha, Yuri S. Berezovsky, Natalya N. Makaryants, Larisa N. Chernousova and Elena E. Larionova

*Address all correspondence to: grand63@yandex.ru

Central TB Research Institute, Moscow, Russia

References

[1] Krasnik M, Vilmann P, Larsen SS, Jacobsen GK. Preliminary experience with a new method of endoscopic transbronchial real time ultrasound guided biopsy for diagnosis of mediastinal and hilar lesions. Thorax. 2003;58(12):1083–6.

[2] Momen M. Wahidi, Felix Herth, Kazuhiro Yasufuku et al. Technical aspects of endobronchial ultrasound-guided transbronchial needle aspiration: CHEST guideline and expert panel report. Chest. 2016;149(3):816–835. doi:10.1378/chest.15-1216

[3] Xiang Y, Zhang F, Akulian J, Yarmus L, Feller-Kopman D, Wang KP. EBUS-TBNA by a new Fuji EBUS scope (with video). J Thorac Dis. 2013;5(1):36–9. doi:10.3978/j.issn. 2072-1439.2012.12.06

[4] Felix J. Herth, Daniela Gompelmann, Pallav L. Shah, Ralf Eberhardt. Endobronchial ultrasound-guided TBNA (EBUS-TBNA) with a 19 gauge needle—first experience. Am J Respir Crit Care Med . 2015;191:A3726.

[5] Detterbeck FC, Lewis S, Diekemper R, Addrizzo-Harris D, Alberts W. Diagnosis and management of lung cancer, 3rd ed: American College of Chest Physicians Evidence-Based Clinical Practice Guidelines. Chest. 2013;143(suppl 5):7S–37S. doi:10.1378/chest. 12-2377.

[6] Vilmann P, Clementsen PF, Colella S et al. Combined endobronchial and oesophageal endosonography for the diagnosis and staging of lung cancer. European Society of Gastrointestinal Endoscopy (ESGE) Guideline, in cooperation with the European Respiratory Society (ERS) and the European Society of Thoracic Surgeons (ESTS). Eur Respir J. 2015;46(1):40–60. doi:10.1183/09031936.00064515

[7] Yasufuku K, Chiyo M, Sekine Y, Chhajed PN et al. Real-time endobronchial ultrasound-guided transbronchial needle aspiration of mediastinal and hilar lymph nodes. Chest. 2004;126:122–128.

[8] Chuchalin AG, Vizel AA et al. Diagnosis and treatment of sarcoidosis: a summary of federal consensus clinical guidelines. Part 2: Diagnosis, treatment, prognosis. Bull Contemp Clin. 2014;7(5):73–81.

[9] Sivokozov I. First experience with the 22 gauge EchoTip ProCore EBUS needle in cases with suspected lymphoma. Channel. 2014;2:12–14.

[10] Fujiwara T, Yasufuku K, Nakajima T et al. The utility of sonographic features during endobronchial ultrasound-guided transbronchial needle aspiration for lymph node staging in patients with lung cancer: a standard endobronchial ultrasound image classification system. Chest. 2010;138(3):641–647. doi:10.1378/chest.09-2006

[11] Nakajima T, Anayama T, Shingyoji M, Kimura H, Yoshino I, Yasufuku K. Vascular image patterns of lymph nodes for the prediction of metastatic disease during EBUS-TBNA

for mediastinal staging of lung cancer. J Thorac Oncol. 2012;7(6):1009–14. doi:10.1097/JTO.0b013e31824cbafa

[12] Saftoiu A, Vilman P. Endoscopic ultrasound elastography—a new imaging technique for the visualization of tissue elasticity distribution. Gastrointestin Liver Dis. 2006;15:161–5.

[13] Trosini-Desert V, Jeny F, Taillade L, Vignot S, Zribi H, Capron F, et al. Bronchial endoscopic ultrasound elastography: preliminary feasibility data. Eur Respir J. 2013;41:477–9.

[14] Izumo T, Sasada S, Chavez C, Matsumoto Y, Tsuchida T. Endobronchial ultrasound elastography in the diagnosis of mediastinal and hilar lymph nodes. Jpn J Clin Oncol. 2014;44(10):956–62. doi:10.1093/jjco/hyu105

[15] Sivokozov IV, Silina TL, Korolev VN et al. The first experience in using elastography in combination with endobronchial ultrasonography for mediastinal pathology: preliminary assessment of feasibility and comparison of characteristics via different approaches. Vestn Rentgenol Radiol. 2014;(4):13–19.

[16] Rozman A, Malovrh MM, Adamic K et al. Endobronchial ultrasound elastography strain ratio for mediastinal lymph node diagnosis. Radiol Oncol. 2015;49(4):334–40. doi: 10.1515/raon-2015-0020

[17] Ishikawa H, Hirooka Y et al. A comparison of image quality between tissue harmonic imaging and fundamental imaging with an electronic radial scanning echoendoscope in the diagnosis of pancreatic diseases. Gastrointest Endosc. 2003;57(7):931–6.

[18] Sung Ill Jang, Dong Ki Lee. Contrast-enhanced endoscopic ultrasonography: advance and current status. Ultrasonography. 2014;33(3):161–169. doi:10.14366/usg.14017

[19] Kanamori A, Hirooka Y, Itoh A et al. Usefulness of contrast-enhanced endoscopic ultrasonography in the differentiation between malignant and benign lymphadenopathy. Am J Gastroenterol. 2006;101(1):45–51.

[20] Oki M, Saka H, Kitagawa C et al. Randomized study of 21-gauge versus 22-gauge endobronchial ultrasound-guided transbronchial needle aspiration needles for sampling histology specimens. J Bronchol Interv Pulmonol. 2011;18:306–310.

[21] Nakajima T,Yasufuku K,Takahashi R et al. Comparison of 21-gauge and 22-gauge aspiration needle during endobronchial ultrasound-guided transbronchial needle aspiration. Respirology. 2011;16:90–94.

[22] Yarmus L.B, Akulian J, Lechtzin N et al. Comparison of 21-gauge and 22-gauge aspiration needle in endobronchial ultrasound-guided transbronchial needle aspiration: results of the American College of Chest Physicians Quality Improvement Registry, Education, and Evaluation Registry. Chest. 2013;143:1036–43.

[23] Jeyabalan A, Shelley-Fraser G, Medford AR. Impact of needle gauge on characterization of endobronchial ultrasound-guided transbronchial needle aspiration (EBUS-TBNA) histology samples. Respirology. 2014;19:735–739.

[24] Izumo T, Sasada S, Watanabe J, Chavez C, Matsumoto Y, Tsuchida T. Comparison of two 22 G aspiration needles for histologic sampling during endobronchial ultrasound-guided transbronchial needle aspiration (EBUS-TBNA). Jpn J Clin Oncol. 2014;44(9): 841–5. doi:10.1093/jjco/hyu095

[25] Xing J, Manos S, Monaco SE, Wilson DO, Pantanowitz L. Endobronchial ultrasound-guided transbronchial needle aspiration: a pilot study to evaluate the utility of the ProCore biopsy needle for lymph node sampling. Acta Cytol. 2016;60(3):254–9.

[26] Sivokozov I, Lovacheva O et al. Comparative efficacy of endoscopic ultrasound-guided fine-needle aspiration for different 22G needle types using bronchoscope in mediastinal lymphadenophaties of uncertain origin. Am J Respir Crit Care. 2014;189:A4403.

[27] Szlubowski A, Kuzdzał J et al. Ultrasound guided transbronchial needle aspiration as a diagnostic tool for lung cancer and sarcoidosis. Pneumonol Alergol Pol. 2008;76(4): 229–36.

[28] Kim JH, Park SW et al. Meta-analysis for Cyto-Pathological outcomes in endoscopic ultrasonography-guided fine-needle aspiration with and without the stylet. Dig Dis Sci. 2016;61(8):2175–84.

[29] van der Heijden EH, Casal R et al. Guideline for the acquisition and preparation of conventional and endobronchial ultrasound-guided transbronchial needle aspiration specimens for the diagnosis and molecular testing of patients with known or suspected lung cancer. Respiration. 2014;88:500–517. doi:10.1159/000368857

[30] Nakajima T, Yasufuku K, Shibuya K, Fujisawa T. Endobronchial ultrasound-guided transbronchial needle aspiration for the treatment of central airway stenosis caused by a mediastinal cyst. Eur J Cardiothorac Surg. 2007;32(3):538–40.

[31] Casal RF, Jimenez CA, Mehran RJ et al. Infected mediastinal bronchogenic cyst successfully treated by endobronchial ultrasound-guided fine-needle aspiration. Ann Thorac Surg. 2010;90(4):e52–3. doi:10.1016/j.athoracsur.2010.06.062.

[32] Maturu VN, Dhooria S, Agarwal R. Efficacy and safety of transbronchial needle aspiration in diagnosis and treatment of mediastinal bronchogenic cysts: systematic review of case reports. J Bronchol Interv Pulmonol. 2015;22(3):195–203. doi:10.1097/ LBR.0000000000000174

[33] Hohenforst-Schmidt W, Zarogoulidis P, Brachmann J et al. Intratumoral chemotherapy for lung cancer: re-challenge current targeted therapies. Drug Des Dev Ther. 2013;18(7): 571–83. doi:10.2147/DDDT.S46393

[34] Mehta HJ, Begnaud A, Penley AM et al. Treatment of isolated mediastinal and hilar recurrence of lung cancer with bronchoscopic endobronchial ultrasound guided intratumoral injection of chemotherapy with cisplatin. Lung Cancer. 2015;90(3):542–7. doi:10.1016/j.lungcan.2015.10.009

[35] von Bartheld MB, van Breda A, Annema JT. Complication rate of endosonography (endobronchial and endoscopic ultrasound): a systematic review. Respiration. 2014;87:343–351.

[36] Agarwal R, Srinivasan A, Aggarwal AN, Gupta D. Efficacy and safety of convex probe EBUS-TBNA in sarcoidosis: a systematic review and meta-analysis. Respir Med. 2012;106(6):883–92.

[37] Evison M, Crosbie PA, Martin J, Bishop P, Doran H, Joseph L, Chaturvedi A, Barber PV, Booton R. EBUS-TBNA in elderly patients with lung cancer: safety and performance outcomes. J Thorac Oncol. 2014;9(3):370–6.

[38] Li W, Zhang T, Chen Y, Liu C, Peng W2. Diagnostic value of convex probe endobronchial ultrasound-guided transbronchial needle aspiration in mediastinal tuberculous lymphadenitis: a systematic review and meta-analysis. Med Sci Monit. 2015;16(21): 2064–72.

[39] Ye W, Zhang R, Xu X, Liu Y, Ying K. Diagnostic efficacy and safety of endobronchial ultrasound-guided transbronchial needle aspiration in intrathoracic tuberculosis: a meta-analysis. J Ultrasound Med. 2015;34(9):1645–50.

[40] Trisolini R, Lazzari Agli L, Tinelli C, De Silvestri A, Scotti V, Patelli M. Endobronchial ultrasound-guided transbronchial needle aspiration for diagnosis of sarcoidosi7s in clinically unselected study populations. Respirology. 2015;20(2):226–34. doi:10.1111/resp.12449

[41] Kheir F, Itani A, Assasa O, Alraiyes AH. The utility of endobronchial ultrasound-transbronchial needle aspiration in lymphoma. Endosc Ultrasound. 2016;5(1):43–48. doi:10.4103/2303-9027.175884.

Chapter 4

Endoluminal Ultrasonography of the Rectum and the Anal Canal

Lidia Ciobanu and Radu Badea

Additional information is available at the end of the chapter

http://dx.doi.org/10.5772/66081

Abstract

Ultrasonography of the anal canal, the rectum and the surrounding tissues using intraluminal transducers with transanal/rectal imaging provides high-resolution imaging with clearly distinguishable tissue-dependent echo signals. Endorectal ultrasonography depicts rectal wall layers and adjuvant structures with a high degree of precision. Anal endosonography is carried out to examine the sphincter muscles and the pelvic floor.

Detailed ultrasonographic anatomy is presented. Specific information is noted regarding the use of radial and linear scanning. The Doppler techniques depict the vascularization. Contrast-enhanced harmonic imaging and elastography are discussed in an integrative manner regarding their role in differentiating malignant from benign ano-rectal masses or lymph nodes. Three-dimensional endorectal ultrasonography provides superior visual images of tumor volume and the spatial relationships of tumor to surrounding anatomical structures.

Endorectal ultrasonography technique accurately measures the size, circumference and distance of the tumor from various anatomic landmarks. It is capable of examining the anal sphincters for tumor infiltration, allowing the surgeon to decide whether a sphincter-sparing resection might be indicated. It can depict the relationship of tumor the to the pelvic peritoneal reflection, to determine whether local excision is possible.

Endorectal ultrasonography in benign pathology is emphasized.

Brief conclusions are given at the end of the chapter.

Keywords: endoluminal ultrasonography, rectum, anal canal, endorectal ultrasonography, anorectal cancer, rectal benign pathology

1. Introduction

The anorectal pathology is very frequent in clinical practice, the patients being addressed for anal fistula, fecal incontinence, hemorrhoidal disease, anal pain, anal fissure, rectocele, rectal prolapse, and rectal tumor. After the clinical and digital rectal exam, the ultrasonography represents the next step in the diagnostic procedure. To obtain reliable details, the transducers have to be as close to the organ of interest as possible. The conventional ultrasound of this region has several limitations considering the position of these organs in the pelvic cavity. The first ultrasound images of the bowel wall using an ultrasound transducer inside a body cavity were obtained in 1950 by Wild [1]. Nowadays the technical improvements of endorectal sonography provide very precise details of rectal wall layers and adjuvant structures, including the pelvic organs. There are two main approaches with corresponding equipment:

- Anorectal ultrasonography performed by clinicians and radiologists
- Endoscopic ultrasound using flexible endoscope-mounted systems performed by gastroenterologists

Understanding the anatomy of the anorectal region and the main clinical indications remain the cornerstone for this examination, independent of the approach and equipment.

2. Anatomy of the anorectal region

The rectum is the final part of the large intestine, which is about 12–14 cm long and has a diameter of 2–6 cm, related to the content [2]. It begins at the rectosigmoid junction, at the level of the third sacral vertebra and runs inferiorly along the curve of the sacrum to pass through the pelvic diaphragm, where it is continued with the anal canal [3]. The rectum is surrounded by fatty tissue that contains blood vessels, nerves, lymphatics, and small lymph nodes [3]. It is delineated posterior by sacro-coccygeal bone structure, inferior by the insertion of the levator ani muscles and superior by the peritoneum [2]. The superior one-third is covered anteriorly and laterally by the pelvic peritoneum. The middle one-third is covered with peritoneum only anteriorly, which curves onto the bladder in the male and onto the uterus in the female. The lower one-third lacks of peritoneum and is related anteriorly to the bladder base, ureters, seminal vesicles, and prostate in the male and to the lower uterus, cervix, and vagina in the female [3].

The internal sphincter, the longitudinal muscle layer, and the external sphincter surround the anal canal. It is delineated posterior by the levator ani muscles, laterally by the ischioanal fossa, and anterior by the apex of the prostate and the membranous urethra in male and posterior wall of the vagina in female [2, 3].

The sphincter anal complex is formed by the muscles that represent the continuation of circular layer of the muscularis propria of the rectum, the striated external anal sphincter, and puborectal muscles, which belong to the levator ani muscles [4]. The lowest point of the external anal sphincter represents the upper anal margin; it is called the anal verge and is the principal landmark for rectal measurements [4]. The pectinate (dentate) line is located 1.5–2 cm upwards from the anus and separates the canal anal into the anatomical part located below the line and the surgical part located above the line [4]. The surgical anal canal extends from the pectinate line to the level of the puborectalis sling, which corresponds to the anorectal junction. The pectinate line is not detectable on radiological studies, representing the endoscopic view of the demarcation between the squamous epithelium (anoderm) and the columnar epithelium [4]. The anoderm is directly attached to the internal anal sphincter [4].

The mesorectum is represented by the connective tissue, located between the middle part of the rectum and the upper surface of the levator ani. The mesorectum contains lymph nodes and neurovascular bundles, fat and fibrous tissue. It is limited posterolaterally by the pelvic visceral fascia and ventrally by an upper continuation of the rectogenital membrane (Denonvilliers' fascia). In females, this dense band forms the rectovaginal septum and in males, the rectoprostatic fascia. Laterally a tiny structure is detected, known as mesorectal or perirectal fascia [4].

The rectal vascularization is provided by the rectal arteries (superior rectal artery from the inferior mesenteric artery, middle rectal artery from the internal iliac artery, and inferior rectal artery from the internal pudendal artery). The rectal venous drainage is realized by the superior rectal vein (that drains into the inferior mesenteric vein) and by the middle and inferior rectal veins (that drains into the iliac veins) [2].

The lymphatic drainage is realized into three circuits:

1. superior station—drains the lymph vessels corresponding to the inferior mesenteric vessels and superior rectal vessels. This circuit has intermediate lymph nodes localized posteriorly and laterally to the rectum.
2. middle station—drains the lymph vessels into the iliac lymph nodes.
3. inferior station—drains the lymph vessels into the superficial inguinal lymph nodes [2].

Ultrasonography of the anal canal, the rectum, and the surrounding tissues using intraluminal transducers with transanal/rectal imaging provides high-resolution imaging with clearly distinguishable tissue-dependent echo signals. Endorectal sonography is able to depict the rectal wall layers and the adjuvant structures, including the pelvic organs with a high degree of precision. Anal endosonography is carried out to examine the sphincter muscles and the pelvic floor.

3. Techniques and procedures used in endorectal ultrasonography

3.1. Conventional 2D ultrasound examination

The endoluminal ultrasonography is highly effective in most cases of anorectal pathology, as it provides accurate evaluation of rectal, perirectal, anal, and perianal pathology. It might be performed without preparation, but an enema significantly improves the image quality, especially in the oncological patients with stool residues [5]. The examination is carried out in the left recumbent position. In patients with sphincter insufficiency, the knee-elbow position might be preferred [4].

The endoluminal ultrasound examination is mandatorily done after digital rectal exam and preferred after a proctoscopy examination. In case of an anal stricture, an inserted finger can appreciate the possible passage of the probe.

A mechanical or a biplanar transducer with a frequency of 10 MHz or higher is most frequently used [2, 4, 5]. Higher frequencies provide better resolution of the rectal wall and sphincter complex, while lower ones depict better, the components of the mesorectum [4].

A condom containing gel is placed over the probe and a thin layer of water-soluble lubricant is placed on the exterior of the condom [3]. The transducer is inserted in a blind gentle manner and the patient is informed about the potential discomfort or pain during the examination [2].

Some authors advice using a 3D 16 MHz probe for the spatial analysis of both the rectum and the surrounding tissues [6].

By convention, the transducer is placed to provide the following image: the anterior aspect of the anal canal will be at 12 o'clock on the screen, right lateral will be at 9 o'clock, left lateral will be at 3 o'clock and posterior will be at 6 o'clock [3]. The depiction of all layers is possible for the whole circumference of the anal canal. At the origin of the anal canal, the "U" shape of the puborectalis sling is the main landmark and must be always identified [3].

Five hypoechoic and hyperechoic layers are depicted corresponding to the anal canal wall [7, 8]. These five identified layers, from inner to outer are:

- the first hyperechoic layer corresponds to the interface between the transducer and the anal mucosal surface,
- the second hypoechoic layer is represented by the subepithelial tissues, being moderately reflective. The mucosa and the dental line are not identified by endoluminal ultrasound,
- the third hypoechoic layer corresponds to the internal sphincter, which is not completely symmetric, either in thickness or termination. It is continued superiorly with the circular muscle of the rectum. In elderly, this layer is inhomogeneous and more echoic [8],
- the fourth hyperechoic layer represents the longitudinal muscle, without constant thickness along the entire anal canal. The increased fibrous stroma is responsible for the echoic aspect of this smooth muscle. In the inter-sphincterian space, the longitudinal muscle and the striated muscles fibers from the levator ani forms "conjoined longitudinal layer" [9],
- the fifth mixed echoic layer corresponds to the external anal sphincter; it has three parts [10]: (1) – the deep part contains the puborectalis muscle, (2) the superficial part has a broad attachment to the underside of the coccyx via the anococcygeal ligament. (3) the subcutaneous part lies below the internal sphincter.

In the axial plane, the upper part of the anal canal corresponds to the puborectalis muscle sling, the deep part of the external anal sphincter, and the complete ring of the internal anal sphincter. The middle part of the anal canal is formed by the superficial part of the external anal sphincter, the conjoined longitudinal layer, the complete ring of the internal anal sphincter, and the transverse perinea muscles. The lower part of the anal canal contains the subcutaneous components of the external anal sphincter [7].

For the rectal examination, especially in oncological patients, special water-filled balloons might be used (**Figure 1**). These balloons filled with about 90 ml of water compress the lesions and remove air from the rectum [5].

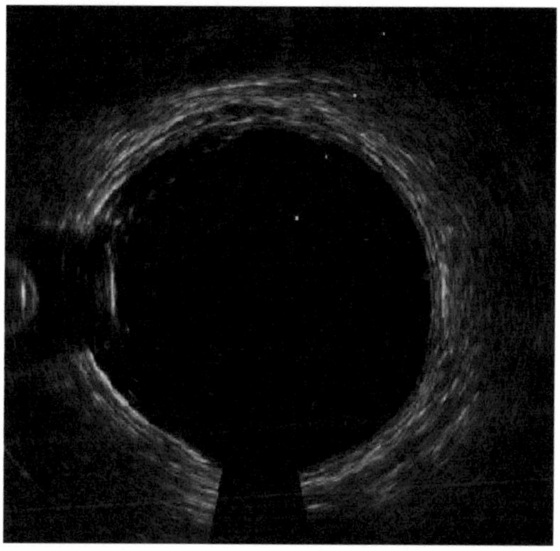

Figure 1. Endocavitary rectal examination – special water filled balloon.

The rectal wall consists of five layers surrounded by perirectal fat or serosa, measuring 2–3 mm. The five layers represent (**Figure 2**) [3]:

- the first hyperechoic layer depicts the interface between the balloon/transducer and the mucosal surface
- the second hypoechoic layer corresponds to the mucosa and the muscularis mucosa,
- the third hyperechoic layer represents the submucosa the fourth hypoechoic layer identifies the muscularis propria
- the fifth hyperechoic layer corresponds to the serosa or to the interface with the mesorectum. The mesorectum has an inhomogeneous pattern due to mixed anatomical structures: blood vessels, nerves, and lymphatic vessels.

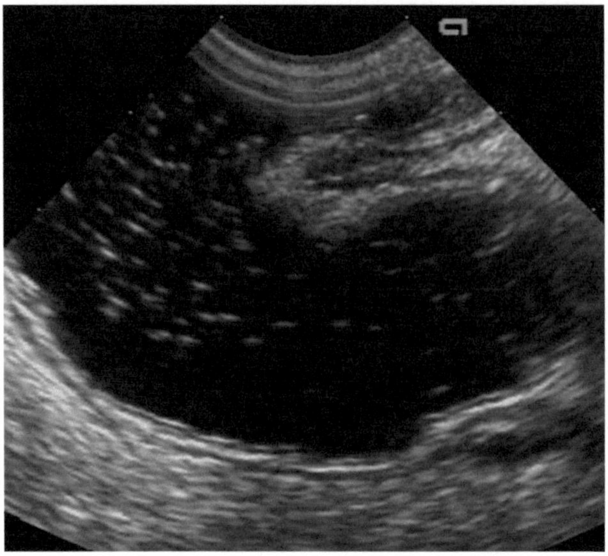

Figure 2. The rectal wall consists of five layers surrounded by perirectal fat or serosa.

Depending on the position of the probe, the surrounding muscles are identified. The external anal sphincter is detected in the lower third of the rectum. Slightly above, it is replaced by the fibers corresponding to the levator ani muscles, that form puborectalis muscle sling. Between the puborectalis muscle sling and caudally located external sphincter, there is an intersphincterian plane filled with the lowest, tapered part of the mesorectum [11]. This plane is important for surgery and for the staging of the anal cancer [11].

Endorectal ultrasound provides an accurate visualization of all pelvic organs adjacent to the rectum: the bladder, the intestinal loops, the seminal vesicles, and prostate in males, and the uterus, cervix, vagina, and urethra in females [3].

The endoscopic approach is nowadays frequently used by the gastroenterologist to assess the anorectal region by ultrasound. Initially, the standard radial endoscopic ultrasound scan was used. The rigid endoscopic ultrasound scan has been used since the early 1980s. Technical improvements provided different types of linear as well as radial scanning devices with frequency varying from 5 MHz to 15 MHz [12]. The echoendoscope is inserted and advanced beyond the lesion, under direct visualization to the rectosigmoid junction. The balloon is slowly inflated and the lumen is filled with water. From this position in the middle of the lumen, the scope is to achieve perpendicular imaging of the rectal wall layers. Once the bladder is identified, the image is mechanically rotated so the bladder is located at 12 o'clock position. Then the instrument is withdrawn slowly, with the transducer kept at the middle of the rectum. No torching of the instrument is recommended, as this causes tangential imaging and possible inaccurate assessment of the depth of tumor penetration. In males, upon withdrawing the probe at 12 o'clock position, the seminal vesicles and the prostate are displayed. In females, this manoeuvre brings in view the uterus and then the vagina, with a hyperechoic band in the center that represents air [13].

http://dx.doi.org/10.5772/66081

3.2. Contrast endoluminal ultrasonography of the rectum and the anal canal

Different ultrasound techniques improve daily practice in benign and malignant pathology. Local contrast agents facilitate the depiction of fistulas through direct administration (**Figure 3**). Intravenous contrast agents define vascular pattern for tumor pathology related to anorectal region or prostate (**Figure 4**).

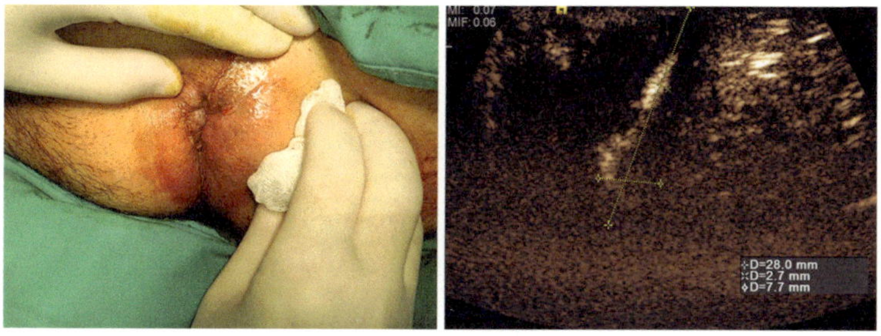

Figure 3. (a) Anal fistula—physical exam. (b) Local contrast agent (Sonovue in this particular case) was administered through the external end of the fistula for better delineation of the size and fistula tract.

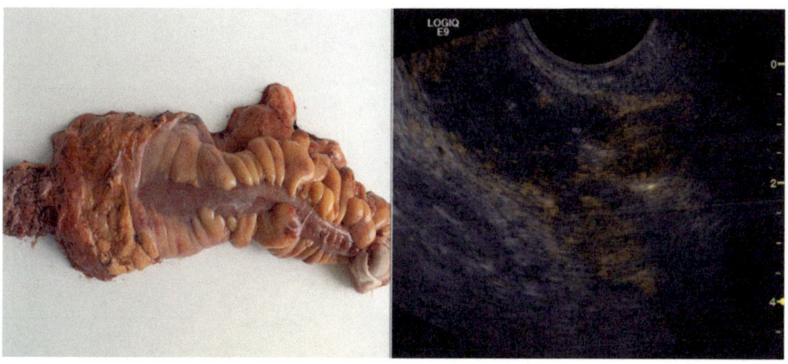

Figure 4. (a) Anorectal tumor—surgically removed. (b) Intravenous contrast agents (Sonovue) was administered. In the venous phase, the contrast agent was washed-out from the tumor (becoming hypoechoic), permitting a better delinia-tion of the tumor from the adjacent organs.

Hydrogen peroxide was investigated as an image-enhancing contrast agent for improving the depiction and the characterization of the fistulas during endoanal ultrasonography [14]. After a conventional endoanal ultrasound is performed, external perianal openings are cannulated and approximately 1 ml of peroxide is administered. After reinsertion of the endoprobe, the entire course of the echogenic fistula, including its relation to the internal and external sphincters and the levator ani muscle are depicted in real time, which facilitates surgical planning [14].

The use of contrast agents within the bloodstream gained more and more applications in the last few years, as it enables the detection of very slow blood flow in vessels measuring as little as 40 μm. Contrast enhanced ultrasound (CEUS) provides valuable information regarding the characterization of a circulatory bed and the evaluation of the neoangiogenesis process [15]. Quantitative parameters are determined during the passage of the contrast agents through a region of interest, mainly by analysis of the time-intensity curve parameters [15]. For rectal cancer, CEUS provides noninvasive biomarkers of tumor angiogenesis and might predict patient prognosis [16]. Contrast enhanced endorectal sonography increases the detection of prostate cancer and facilitates the target biopsies [17, 18].

3.3. Doppler ultrasonography

The Doppler ultrasonography provides information regarding the flow within large vessels. Doppler-guided hemorrhoidal ligation was introduced into clinical practice 20 years ago (**Figure 5**) [19]. Doppler-guided hemorrhoidal dearterialization is a safe and effective method to treat grades II–IV hemorrhoidal diseases, especially in those with previous anal surgeries or previous alterations of fecal continence, when an additional procedure might represent a risk of definitive incontinence [19].

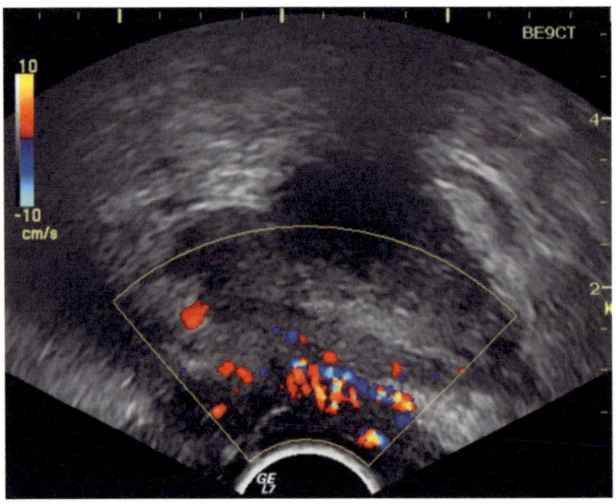

Figure 5. Doppler ultrasonography provides information regarding the flow within large vessels in the anorectal region.

3.4. Transanal real-time elastography

The transanal real-time elastage in rectal cancer ranges is between 80stography was demonstrated to yield valuable information regarding elastic properties of the anal sphincter, especially in patients with fecal incontinence. A pathological elastogram is considered, when predominantly hard elements are detected. This technique was investigated in different pathologies, anorectal surgery in irradiated and non-irradiated individuals and Crohn's disease. Based on studies conducted by Allgayer et al. [20, 21] the transanal real-time elastography with quantitation of sphincter elastic properties yields no further diagnostic and prognostic information compared to conventional endosonography.

3.5. Three-dimensional ultrasound

The three-dimensional ultrasound is provided from the synthesis of a high number of parallel transaxial two-dimensional images [3]. The image can be rotated, tilted, and sliced to allow the physician to analyze different section parameters, different angles and to assess accurately distances, areas, angles, and volumes [3]. Three-dimensional endorectal ultrasonography is useful for assessing the depth of submucosal invasion in early rectal cancer and for selecting therapeutic options [22].

4. Endorectal ultrasonography examination for diagnosis and staging of rectal and anal tumors

The management of patients with anorectal neoplasm requires specific information regarding:

- tumor spread (T features),
- detailed evaluation of mesorectal fascia,
- extramural venous invasion,
- lymph nodes involvement (N features),
- presence of distance metastasis (M features) [4].

The tumor-node-metastasis (TNM) system represents the standard of care for rectal and anal staging (**Table 1**) [23].

The ultrasound feature of rectal cancer is a hypoechoic lesion that disrupts the normal five-layer sonographic structures of the rectal wall. The distal border of the tumor must be precisely depicted in relation to the anterior peritoneal reflection (in males, the relation of the distal border of the tumor to the seminal vesicles and in females, to the cervix are determined) [24].

The ultrasound images relevant to T staging are:

- T_{is} corresponds to the first hypoechoic layer expended, but without the second hyperechoic layer involvement.
- T_1 invades the submucosa, but without muscularis propria involvement, it is detected in ultrasound when the second hyperechoic layer is stippled or broken in appearance, but generally intact.
- T_2 ultrasound appearance is depicted when the second hyperechoic layer is completely disrupted and the mass may extend into the second hypoechoic layer.
- T_3 corresponds to the perirectal fat or serosa invasion, the outer hyperechoic layer is disrupted.
- T_4 is easy diagnosed as the tumor is extended into neighboring organs [25].

	Anal carcinoma	Rectal carcinoma
T_x	Primary tumor cannot be assessed	Primary tumor cannot be assessed
T_0	No evidence of primary tumor	No evidence of primary tumor
T_{is}	Carcinoma *in situ*, Bowen disease, high grade squamous intraepithelial lesion (HSIL), anal intraepithelial neoplasia II-III (AIN II-III)	Carcinoma *in situ*: intraepithelial or invasion of lamina propria
T_1	Tumor 2 cm or less in the greatest dimension	Tumor invades submucosa
T_2	Tumor more than 2 cm, but not more than 5 cm in the greatest dimension	Tumor invades muscularis propria
T_3	Tumor more than 5 cm in the greatest dimension	Tumor invades subserosa or into non-peritonealized perirectal tissues
T_4	Tumor of any size invades adjacent organ(s) (e.g., vagina, urethra, bladder)	Tumor perforates visceral peritoneum (T_{4a}) and/or directly invades other organs or structures (T_{4b})
N_x	Regional lymph node cannot be assessed	Regional lymph node cannot be assessed
N_0	No regional lymph node metastasis	No regional lymph node metastasis
N_1	Metastasis in the perirectal lymph nodes	Metastasis in 1 to 3 regional lymph nodes N_{1a} – Metastasis in 1 regional lymph node N_{1b} – Metastasis in 2–3 regional lymph nodes N_{1c} – Tumor deposit(s), i.e., satellites in the subserosa or in nonperitonalized pericolic or perirectal soft tissue without regional lymph node metastasis
N_2	Metastasis in unilateral internal iliac and/or inguinal lymph nodes	Metastasis in 4 or more regional lymph nodes N_{2a} – metastasis in 4–6 regional lymph nodes N_{2b} – metastasis in more regional lymph nodes
N_3	Metastasis in perirectal and inguinal lymph nodes and/or bilateral internal iliac and/or bilateral inguinal lymph nodes	
M_0	No distal metastasis	No distal metastasis
M_1	Distal metastasis	M_{1a} – metastasis confined to one organ M_{1b} – metastasis in more than one organ or the peritoneum

Table 1. TNM staging principle for the anal and rectal carcinoma according to the current classification of International Agency for Research on Cancer/World Health Organization [23].

The accuracy of T stage in rectal cancer ranges is between 80 and 95% [26, 27]. The T_2 tumors are frequently over-staged as T_3 tumors, because peritumoral inflammation cannot be accurate differentiated from desmoplastic reaction [28]. From the clinical point of view, this overstaging has no significant impact as T_2 tumors have the same prognosis as T_3 tumors with less than 1 mm spread [4] (**Figure 6**). The assessment of T_3 tumors is very important, especially the measurement of the depth of extramural spread in the mesorectal fat, since T_3 tumors with less than 5mm mesorectal invasion have a 5-year survival rate of 85% and T_3 tumors with more than 5 mm mesorectal invasion have a 5-year survival rate of 54% [4, 29, 30]. Minimally invasive T_3 tumors present an invasion into the mesorectal fat less than 2 mm beyond the muscularis propria and advanced T_3 tumor is characterized by an invasion of more than 3 mm [24]. These measurements are difficult to be performed in lower anal canal tumors, on its anterior wall or in patients with a small amount of perirectal fat [4]. The endoscopic ultrasound sensitivity for T stage is highest for advanced disease (96.4% for T_3 and 95.4% for T_4) compared to early disease (87.8% for T_1 and 80.5% for T_2) [31].

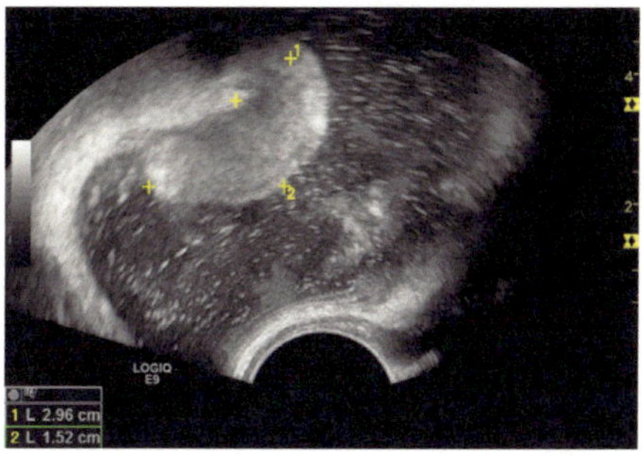

Figure 6. Rectal tumor staging. T_3 corresponds to the perirectal fat or serosa invasion, the outer hyperechoic layer is disrupted.

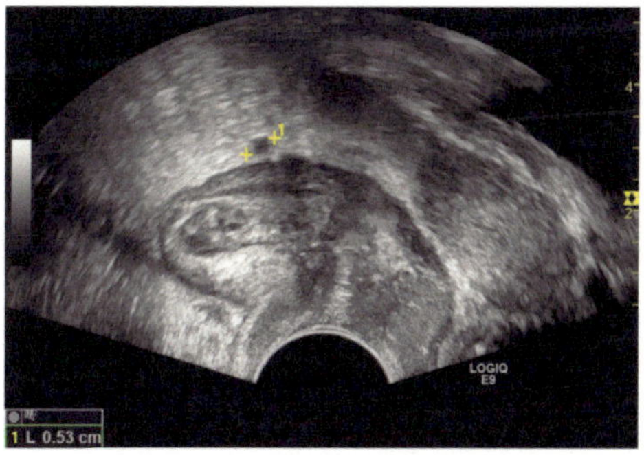

Figure 7. Rectal tumor staging T_3. A round hypoechoic lymph node, measuring 5 mm is detected.

The extramural venous invasion is detected by magnetic resonance imaging using a score proposed by Smith et al. [32] and represents an important prognostic factor since the detected venous invasion had a 3.7 times increased relative risk of metachronous metastatic disease [33].

The assessment of lymph node in patients with rectal cancer represents a debated issue. The ultrasound defines the size, border, shape, and echogenicity and enables tissue biopsy sampling. The features suggestive for malignancies are: enlarged nodes (≥1 cm in short axis), hypoechoic appearance, round shape, and smooth border (**Figures 7** and **8**) [24]. As the accuracy of the endocavitary ultrasound for N stage is moderate [31], fine needle aspiration should be used when critical decision regarding neo-adjuvant chemotherapy is proposed [24].

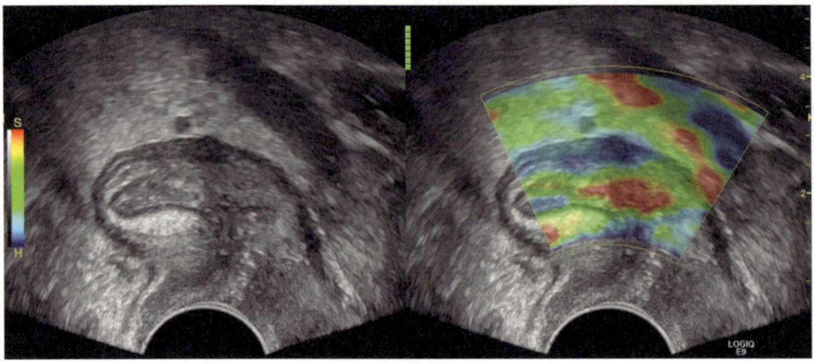

Figure 8. Rectal tumor. 2D ultrasound image and elastography. The rectal tumor is depicted stiffer than the tumor-free rectal wall and the perirectal fat tissue (colored in blue).

Different new ultrasound techniques has improved the diagnosis of the rectal and anal canal tumors.

3D-endocavitary ultrasound allows an accurate measurement of rectal tumors and identification of anatomical relationships, which assists the surgical planning procedure (**Figure 9**).

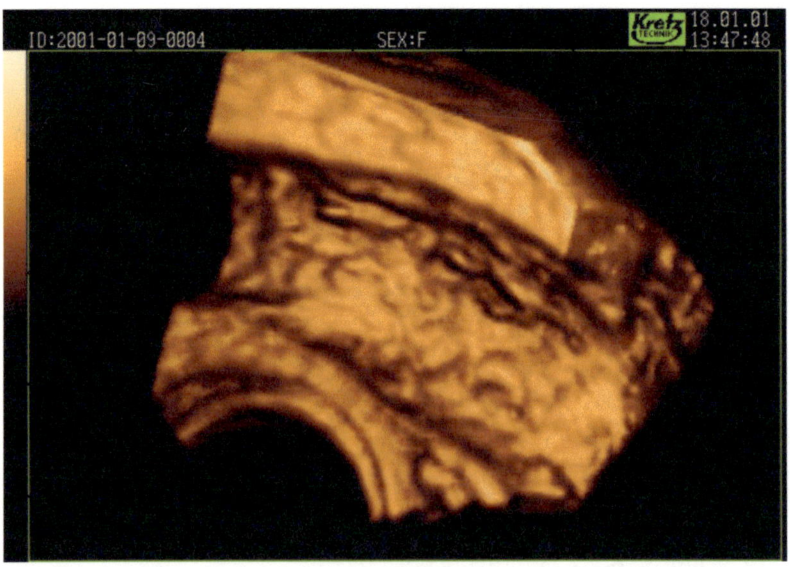

Figure 9. 3D endocavitary ultrasound offers a spatial assessment of the rectal tumor.

Contrast enhanced ultrasound depicts the vascular pattern for rectal lesions [15]. Quantitative parameters might be measured during the passage of the contrast agents through a region of interest, mainly by analysis of the time-intensity curve parameters [15]. For rectal cancer, CEUS provides noninvasive biomarkers of the neoangiogenesis and might predict patient prognosis (**Figure 10**) [16].

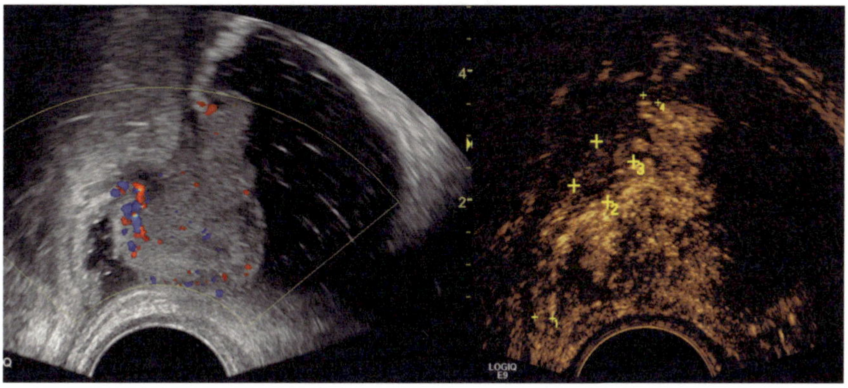

Figure 10. Contrast enhanced ultrasound (Sonovue administered intravenously) depicts the vascular pattern for rectal lesions.

The elastography become an "extension" of the clinical sense, strengthening and confirming the final diagnosis by its ability to measure the tissue elasticity. Different techniques are used: strain elastography imaging (SEI), shear wave imaging (acoustic radiation force impulse imaging (ARFI) and shear wave elasticity imaging (SWEI). ARFI and SWEI are quantitative methods. No data have been published so far concerning their use in the assessment of the rectal tumors. The rectal tumors are stiffer than the tumor-free rectal wall and the perirectal fat tissue. An optimal differentiation between benign and malignant lesions was obtained at a cut-off value of the mean strain ratio cut-off value of 1.25 [34] (**Figures 11** and **12**).

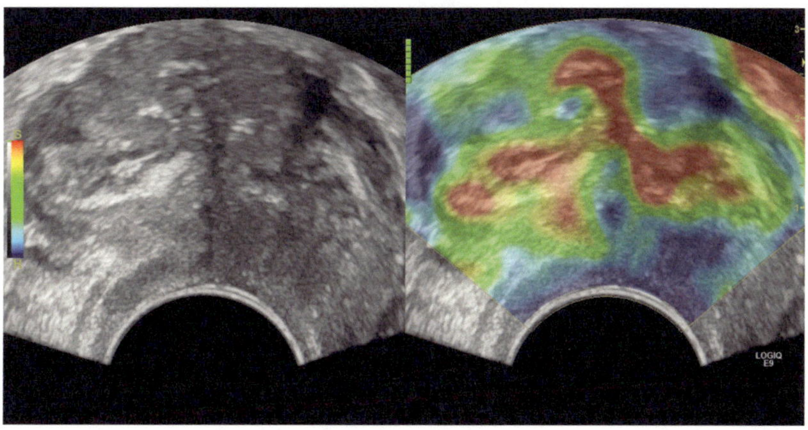

Figure 11. Rectal tumor. 2D ultrasound image and elastography. The rectal tumor is depicted stiffer than the tumor-free rectal wall and the perirectal fat tissue (colored in blue).

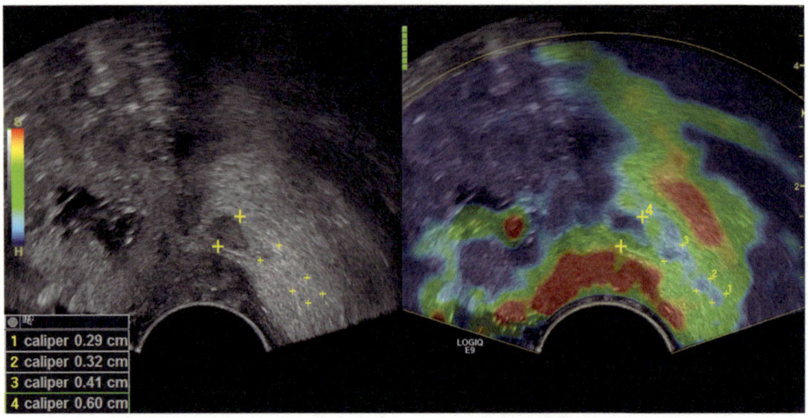

Figure 12. Lymph nodes involvement in a rectal tumor. 2D ultrasound image and elastography. The elastography identifies more malignant lymph nodes than detected by 2D ultrasound (stiffer than the tumor-free rectal wall and the perirectal fat tissue – colored in blue).

Preoperative neoadjuvant chemo-radiotherapy (N_{3-4} or lymph nodes involvement) is used to downstage rectal cancer in order to improve survival and to allow sphincter-preserving low anterior resection [12]. Considering the necrosis, inflammation, and fibrotic changes following neoadjuvant therapy, the assessment of tumor nodes through ultrasound might not be adequate. The T re-stage accuracy is 50% (**Figure 13**) [35–38]. The accuracy can be improved by depicting the intense and chaotic vasculature of residual tumor tissue through Doppler technique [39] or contrast-enhance ultrasound [40, 41].

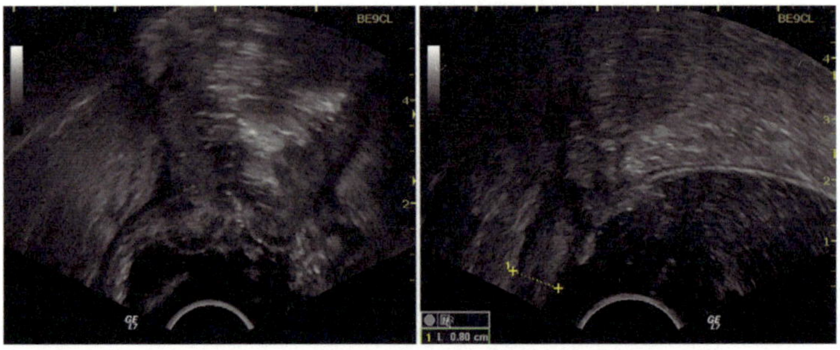

Figure 13. Rectal tumor. (a) In diagnosis the tumor was assessed as T3, invading the perirectal fat. (b) After neoadjuvant radiochemotherapy the tumor decreased in size (8 mm), but still invaded the perirectal fat.

Endoscopic ultrasonography of rectum can also be used for rectal cancer recurrence postoperatively with high accuracy [41, 42]. In some cases the ultrasound feature of tumor recurrence cannot be differentiate by post-surgery fibrosis or inflammation [24]. Obtaining biopsy samples through fine needle aspiration improves the detection of rectal recurrences. Also depiction of the vascularization through Doppler techniques or CEUS can considerably increase the specificity of transrectal ultrasound in differentiating tumor relapse from fibrosis

[39, 40, 43]. The endoscopic ultrasound is recommended for follow up after surgery at six months interval for two years [24]. The anastomotic sites might be revealed as cystic lesions with heterogeneous wall thickening and fine needle aspiration might detect mucin containing inflammatory cells in the absence of malignant cells [44].

5. Endorectal ultrasonography for benign pathology

5.1. Fecal incontinence

Patients with fecal incontinence frequently associate anal sphincter injury as a consequence of obstetrical trauma, anorectal surgery or accidental injury [45]. Endoanal ultrasonography can accurate depict the anal sphincter complex and surrounding perirectal tissues [45]. Anal sphincter tears are depicted as a discontinuity of the hypoechoic structure corresponding to the internal anal sphincter or of the more heterogeneous external anal sphincter [46]. Obstetric injury is located anterior and frequently involves both sphincters [46]. The accuracy of endoanal ultrasound for sphincters disruption is very high: 95% [47, 48].

5.2. Anal fistulae and abscesses

The main causes for anal fistulae and abscesses are: Crohn's disease, post-operative infection, radiotherapy. The Parks classification of perianal fistulae depicts four types: inter, trans, extra and suprasphincterian [49], according to their extension to the external anal sphincter and to the puborectalis muscles. The ultrasound appearance of the fistula is a hypoechoic linear structure with possible hyperechoic reflections (air) between anal canal or rectum or vagina. The use of hydrogen peroxide-enhanced anal endosonography provides better depiction of fistula and its relation to the internal and external sphincters and the levator ani muscles [50]. Alternative to hydrogen peroxide are represented by the new ultrasound contrast agents: Levovist or SonoVue [51]. The sonographic appearance of the abscess is a mass either anechoic or hypoechoic (with internal echoes corresponding to tissue debris) [52]. This technique is recommended for fistula diagnosis and monitoring in patients with Crohn's disease. The use of contrast agents and 3D techniques provides accurate assessment of complex fistula mapping before planning medical or surgery treatment. Also, it is useful for puncturing the abscesses in the operating room using an echoendoscopic approach or a surgery technique [52].

6. Conclusions

Endoluminal ultrasonography of the rectum and the anal canal is a valuable method for the assessment and staging of rectal and anal canal tumors. It is also frequently used for perianal fistulae mapping, anal sphincter tears depiction in patients with fecal incontinence and for abscesses identification and puncturing. Different ultrasound techniques provide morphological, functional and vascular pattern accurate assessment of rectal tumors before surgery, after radiotherapy/chemotherapy, and after surgery (for the detection of relapses).

Author details

Lidia Ciobanu* and Radu Badea

*Address all correspondence to: lidia.ciobanu@umfcluj.ro

University of Medicine and Pharmacy Iuliu Hațieganu, Regional Institute of Gastroenterology and Hepatology, Cluj-Napoca, Romania

References

[1] Wild JJ. The use of ultrasonic pulses for the measurement of biologic tissues and the detection of tissue density changes. Surgery 1950;27:183–188.

[2] Badea R, Dumitrascu DL. The digestive tract. In Badea R, Dudea SM, Mircea PA, Stamatian F, editors. Clinic Ultrasonography Compendium. Medical Publisher, Bucharest 2004. pp. 274–349 [Romanian].

[3] Santoro GA, Di Falco G. Endoanal and endorectal ultrasonography: methodology and normal pelvic floor anatomy. In Santoro GA, Wieczorek AP, Bartram CI, editors. Pelvic Floor Disorders. Spinger-Verlag, Italy 2010. pp. 91–102.

[4] Burdan F, Sudol-Szopinska I, Staroslawska E, Kolodziejczak M, Klepacz R, Mocarska A, Caban M, Zelazowska-Cieslinska I, Szumilo J. Magnetic resonance imaging and endorectal ultrasound for diagnosis of rectal lesions. Eur J Med Res. 2015;20:4. DOI: 10.1186/s40001-014-0078-0.

[5] Sudol-Szopinska I. Endosconograpic examination of the anal canal and rectum. In Jakubowski W, editor. Principles for ultrasound examination. Roztoczanska Szkola Ultrasonografii, Zamosc 2011. pp. 140–144.

[6] Sudoł-Szopińska I, Kołodziejczak M, Szopiński TR. The accuracy of a postprocessing technique—volume render mode—in three-dimensional endoanal ultrasonography of anal abscesses and fistulas. Dis Colon Rectum. 2011;54:238–244. DOI: 10.1007/DCR.0b013e3181ff44de.

[7] Santorro GA, Di Falco G. Endosonographic anatomy of the normal anal canal. In Santorro GA, Di Falco G, editors. Benign Anorectal Diseases. Diagnostic with Endoanal and Endorectal Ultrasonography and New Treatment Options. Springer-Verlag, Milan Italy, 2006. pp. 35–54.

[8] Starck M, Bohe M, Fortling B, Valentin L. Endosonography of the anal sphincter in women of different ages and parity. Ultrasound Obstet Gynecol. 2005;25:169–176.

[9] Shafik A. A new concept of the anatomy of the anal sphincter mechanism and the physiology of defecation. III. The longitudinal anal muscle: anatomy and role in anal sphincter mechanism. Invest Urol. 1976;13:271–277.

[10] Shafik A. A new concept of the anatomy of the anal sphincter mechanism and the physiology of defecation. The external anal sphincter: a triple-loop system. Invest Urol. 1975;12:412–419.

[11] Hoeffel C, Mulé S, Laurent V, Bouché O, Volet J, Soyer P. Primary rectal cancer local staging. Diagn Interv Imaging. 2014;95:485–494. DOI: 10.1016/j.diii.2014.03.005.

[12] Giovannini M, Ardizzone S. Anorectal ultrasound for neoplastic and inflammatory lesions. Best Pract Res Clin Gastroenterol. 2006;20:113–135.

[13] Fockens P, Halligan S, Hawes RH, Varadarajulu S. How to perform anorectal EUS. In Hawes RH, Fockens P, Varadarajulu S, editors. Endosonography, Third Edition. Elsevier Saunders, Philadelphia 2015. pp. 257–259.

[14] Kruskal JB, Kane RA, Morrin MM. Peroxide-enhanced anal endosonography: technique, image interpretation, and clinical applications. Radiographics. 2001;21 Spec No:S173–S189.

[15] Badea R, Ciobanu L. Contrast enhanced and Doppler ultrasonography in the characterization of the microcirculation. Expectancies and performances. Med Ultrason. 2012;14:307–317.

[16] Wang Y, Li L, Wang YX, Cui NY, Zou SM, Zhou CW, Jiang YX. Time-intensity curve parameters in rectal cancer measured using endorectal ultrasonography with sterile coupling gels filling the rectum: correlations with tumor angiogenesis and clinicopathological features. Biomed Res Int. 2014;2014:587806. DOI: 10.1155/2014/587806.

[17] Roy C, Buy X, Lang H, Saussine C, Jacqmin D. Contrast enhanced color Doppler endorectal sonography of prostate: efficiency for detecting peripheral zone tumors and role for biopsy procedure. J Urol. 2003;170:69–72.

[18] Mitterberger M, Pinggera GM, Horninger W, Bartsch G, Strasser H, Schäfer G, Brunner A, Halpern EJ, Gradl J, Pallwein L, Frauscher F. Comparison of contrast enhanced color Doppler targeted biopsy to conventional systematic biopsy: impact on Gleason score. J Urol. 2007;178:464–468.

[19] Figueiredo MN, Campos FG. Doppler-guided hemorrhoidal dearterialization/transanal hemorrhoidal dearterialization: Technical evolution and outcomes after 20 years. World J Gastrointest Surg. 2016;8:232–237. DOI: 10.4240/wjgs.v8.i3.232.

[20] Allgayer H, Ignee A, Dietrich CF. Endosonographic elastography of the anal sphincter in patients with fecal incontinence. Scand J Gastroenterol. 2010;45:30–38. DOI: 10.3109/00365520903383251.

[21] Allgayer H, Ignee A, Zipse S, Crispin A, Dietrich CF. Endorectal ultrasound and real-time elastography in patients with fecal incontinence following anorectal surgery: a

prospective comparison evaluating short- and long-term outcomes in irradiated and non-irradiated patients. Z Gastroenterol. 2012;50:1281–1286. DOI: 10.1055/s-0032-1313000.

[22] Santoro GA, Gizzi G, Pellegrini L, Battistella G, Di Falco G. The value of high-resolution three-dimensional endorectal ultrasonography in the management of submucosal invasive rectal tumors. Dis Colon Rectum. 2009;52:1837–1843. DOI: 10.1007/DCR.0b013e3181b16ce9.

[23] Bosman FT, Carneiro F, Hruban RH, Theise ND (Eds.). WHO classification of Tumors of the Digestive Sysytem (International Agency for Research on Cancer) 4th Edition. Lyon, 2010;132,184.

[24] Gleeson FC. EUS in rectal cancer. In Hawes RH, Fockens P, Varadarajulu S, editors. Endosonography, 3rd Edition. Elsevier Saunders, Philadelphia 2015. pp. 260–268.

[25] Edelman BR, Weiser MR. Endorectal ultrasound: its role in the diagnosis and treatment of rectal cancer. Clin Colon Rectal Surg. 2008;21:167–177. DOI: 10.1055/s-2008-1080996.

[26] Kim NK, Kim MJ, Yun SH, Sohn SK, Min JS. Comparative study of transrectal ultrasonography, pelvic computerized tomography, and magnetic resonance imaging in preoperative staging of rectal cancer. Dis Colon Rectum. 1999;42:770–775.

[27] Halefoglu AM, Yildirim S, Avlanmis O, Sakiz D, Baykan A. Endorectal ultrasonography versus phased-array magnetic resonance imaging for preoperative staging of rectal cancer. World J Gastroenterol. 2008;14:3504–3510.

[28] Kauer WK, Prantl L, Dittler HJ, Siewert JR. The value of endosonographic rectal carcinoma staging in routine diagnostics: a 10-year analysis. Surg Endosc. 2004;18:1075–1078.

[29] Pedersen BG, Moran B, Brown G, Blomqvist L, Fenger-Grøn M, Laurberg S. Reproducibility of depth of extramural tumor spread and distance to circumferential resection margin at rectal MRI: enhancement of clinical guidelines for neoadjuvant therapy. AJR Am J Roentgenol. 2011;197:1360–1366. DOI: 10.2214/AJR.11.6508.

[30] Smith N, Brown G. Preoperative staging of rectal cancer. Acta Oncol. 2008;47:20–31.

[31] Puli SR, Bechtold ML, Reddy JB, Choudhary A, Antillon MR, Brugge WR. How good is endoscopic ultrasound in differentiating various T stages of rectal cancer? Meta-analysis and systematic review. Ann Surg Oncol. 2009;16:254–265. DOI: 10.1245/s10434-008-0231-5.

[32] Smith NJ, Barbachano Y, Norman AR, Swift RI, Abulafi AM, Brown G. Prognostic significance of magnetic resonance imaging-detected extramural vascular invasion in rectal cancer. Br J Surg. 2008;95:229–236.

[33] Bugg WG, Andreou AK, Biswas D, Toms AP, Williams SM. The prognostic significance of MRI-detected extramural venous invasion in rectal carcinoma. Clin Radiol. 2014;69:619–623. DOI: 10.1016/j.crad.2014.01.010.

[34] Waage JE, Havre RF, Odegaard S, Leh S, Eide GE, Baatrup G. Endorectal elastography in the evaluation of rectal tumours. Colorectal Dis. 2011;13:1130–1137. DOI: 10.1111/j.1463-1318.2010.02440.x.

[35] Vanagunas A, Lin DE, Stryker SJ. Accuracy of endoscopic ultrasound for restaging rectal cancer following neoadjuvant chemoradiation therapy. Am J Gastroenterol. 2004;99:109–112.

[36] Romagnuolo J, Parent J, Vuong T, Bélanger M, Michel RP, Belliveau PJ, Trudel JL. Predicting residual rectal adenocarcinoma in the surgical specimen after preoperative brachytherapy with endoscopic ultrasound. Can J Gastroenterol. 2004;18:435-440.

[37] Maor Y, Nadler M, Barshack I, Zmora O, Koller M, Kundel Y, Fidder H, Bar-Meir S, Avidan B. Endoscopic ultrasound staging of rectal cancer: diagnostic value before and following chemoradiation. J Gastroenterol Hepatol. 2006;21:454–458.

[38] Tankova LT, Penchev PI, Kovatchki D, Stoilov G, Hadjieva T. Endosonographic assessment of rectal cancer after neoadjuvant radiotherapy. Med Ultrason. 2012;14:19–23.

[39] Badea R, Gersak MM, Dudea SM, Graur F, Hajjar NA, Furcea L. Characterization and staging of rectal tumors: endoscopic ultrasound versus MRI/CT. Pictorial essay. Med Ultrason. 2015;17:241–247. DOI: 10.11152/mu.2013.2066.172.mri.

[40] Gersak MM, Badea R, Graur F, Hajja NA, Furcea L, Dudea SM. Endoscopic ultrasound for the characterization and staging of rectal cancer. Current state of the method. Technological advances and perspectives. Med Ultrason. 2015;17:227–234. DOI: 10.11152/mu.2013.2066.172.gsk.

[41] Novell F, Pascual S, Viella P, Trias M. Endorectal ultrasonography in the follow-up of rectal cancer. Is it a better way to detect early local recurrence? Int J Colorectal Dis. 1997;12:78–81.

[42] de Anda EH, Lee SH, Finne CO, Rothenberger DA, Madoff RD, Garcia-Aguilar J. Endorectal ultrasound in the follow-up of rectal cancer patients treated by local excision or radical surgery. Dis Colon Rectum. 2004;47:818–824.

[43] Drudi FM, Giovagnorio F, Raffetto N, Ricci P, Cascone F, Santarelli M, Trippa F, Passariello R. Transrectal ultrasound color Doppler in the evaluation of recurrence of anal canal cancer. Eur J Radiol. 2003;47:142–148.

[44] Honda K, Akahoshi K, Matsui N, Motomura Y, Kubokawa M, Higuchi N, Endo S, Taki K, Oya M. Role of EUS and EUS-guided FNA in the diagnosis of rectal implantation cyst at an anastomosis site after a previous low anterior resection for a rectal cancer

without evidence of cancer recurrence. Gastrointest Endosc. 2008;68:782–785. DOI: 10.1016/j.gie.2008.05.011.

[45] Saranovic D, Barisic G, Krivokapic Z, Masulovic D, Djuric-Stefanovic A. Endoanal ultrasound evaluation of anorectal diseases and disorders: technique, indications, results and limitations. Eur J Radiol. 2007;61:480–489.

[46] Halligan S. Evaluation of the anal sphincter by anal EUS. In Hawes RH, Fockens P, Varadarajulu S, editors. Endosonography, 3rd Edition. Elsevier Saunders, Philadelphia 2015; pp. 269–281.

[47] Fuchsjäger MH, Maier AG. Imaging fecal incontinence. Eur J Radiol. 2003;47:108–116.

[48] Deen KI, Kumar D, Williams JG, Olliff J, Keighley MR. Anal sphincter defects. Correlation between endoanal ultrasound and surgery. Ann Surg. 1993;218:201–205.

[49] Parks AG, Gordon PH, Hardcastle JD. A classification of fistula-in-ano. Br J Surg. 1976;63:1–12.

[50] Ortiz H, Marzo J, Jiménez G, DeMiguel M. Accuracy of hydrogen peroxide-enhanced ultrasound in the identification of internal openings of anal fistulas. Colorectal Dis. 2002;4:280–283.

[51] Chew SS, Yang JL, Newstead GL, Douglas PR. Anal fistula: Levovist-enhanced endoanal ultrasound: a pilot study. Dis Colon Rectum. 2003;46:377–384.

[52] Giovannini M, Bories E, Moutardier V, Pesenti C, Guillemin A, Lelong B, Delpéro JR. Drainage of deep pelvic abscesses using therapeutic echo endoscopy. Endoscopy. 2003;35:511–514.

Chapter 5

Endoscopic Ultrasound and Intestinal Endometriosis

Lucio Giovanni Battista Rossini,
Juliana Marques Drigo and
Gisele de Fatima Cordeiro Leite

Additional information is available at the end of the chapter

http://dx.doi.org/10.5772/66080

Abstract

Endometriosis is a benign gynecological disease characterized by histological confirmation of the presence of ectopic endometrial glands and/or endometrial stroma. The main clinical gynecologic manifestations include chronic pelvic pain, back pain, menstrual disorders, and infertility. Over 60% of women with endometriosis have chronic intestinal symptoms. Intestinal involvement occurs in up to 12% of patients. Intestinal deep infiltrating endometriosis is defined as the lesion infiltrating at least the muscular layer of the bowel wall. Gynecological pelvic exam is not sufficient for the diagnosis of the location of deeply infiltrating endometriosis. Imaging methods can suggest the diagnosis of endometriosis and help to map the disease. Transrectal ultrasound (TRUS) has been used for more than a decade for the diagnosis and staging of deep endometriosis, providing relevant data for surgical treatment. It is useful to determine the depth of infiltration and the distance from the anal junction. The recent trend is to prefer nodule excision, when feasible, rather than radical digestive resection; therefore, it is important to take into consideration the staging of rectal and sigmoid infiltrating endometriosis in the preoperative clinical evaluation.

Keywords: Endometriosis, endosonography, rectal neoplasm, digestive system surgical procedures, gastrointestinal stromal tumors

1. Introduction

Endometriosis is a benign gynecological disease characterized by histological confirmation of the presence of ectopic endometrial glands and/or endometrial stroma [1].

The disease affects 10% of reproductive-age women, and intestinal involvement occurs in up to 12% of patients. It is a costly chronic disease causing pelvic pain and subfertility [2]. Up to 95%

of intestinal endometriosis is found in the rectum and sigmoid colon. In addition, in 39% of the cases, it may be present in more than one intestinal segment. In 20% of the cases, it can be found isolated [1].

1.1. Pathogenesis

There are three theories that explain the appearance of endometriosis. They are coelomic metaplasia, lymphatic or hematogenous dissemination, and retrograde menstruation, which is the most widespread theory. According to the theory of retrograde menstruation, that is, a physiological event in up to 90% of women, viable endometrial cells of the uterine cavity migrated to the tubes, implanting themselves and developing in several ectopic sites [3].

The rectosigmoid colon acts as an anatomic shelter, housing endometrial cells and preventing them from being cleared by the usual menstrual clearing process within the peritoneal cavity. Endometrial implants trigger an inflammatory response, and eventually, a fibrotic nodule is buried under the peritoneum [4].

1.2. Classification

Intestinal deep infiltrating endometriosis is defined as the lesion infiltrating at least the muscular layer of the bowel wall. The mucosa is infiltrated in less than 5% of intestinal lesions [1, 5].

Outside intestinal wall, deep endometriosis is defined as a solid endometriotic mass situated more than 5mm deep into the peritoneum. According to some experts, endometriotic foci located on the bowel serosa that do not meet these criteria are defined as peritoneal endometriosis rather than bowel endometriosis [4].

In normal female pelvic anatomy, the anterior rectum is apposed to the posterior vagina; this is referred to as the rectovaginal septum. Superior to the rectovaginal septum, the vagina and rectum separate and create a peritoneum-lined space called the posterior pouch of Douglas. The anatomic boundaries of pouch of Douglas are as follows: inferiorly, the rectovaginal septum; laterally, the uterosacral ligaments; anteriorly and superiorly, the posterior vagina, cervix, and uterus; posteriorly, the rectum [4].

The layers of stratification of the intestinal wall and some anatomical pelvic limits are of extreme importance for staging and therapeutic definition of intestinal endometriosis [3].

Based on histological and topographic criteria, Rossini, Ribeiro, and Aoki developed the echologic classification to map pelvic lesions based on endoscopic findings [6].

The authors divide the penetration or the absence of intestinal endometriosis in five stages (T1–T5) (**Figure 1**) and five different topographies to define the site of lesions (L1–L5) (**Figure 2**). To delimit the parietal penetration, the authors used sonographic stratification layers of the normal intestinal wall, described by Uncle Tytgat in 1986. In order to designate the anatomical position of the lesion, the authors used the ratio of local involvement with the uterus, the posterior vaginal fornix, and rectovaginal septum. To indicate that the evaluation is being conducted in a sonographic study of suspected endometriosis lesions, the letters

http://dx.doi.org/10.5772/66080

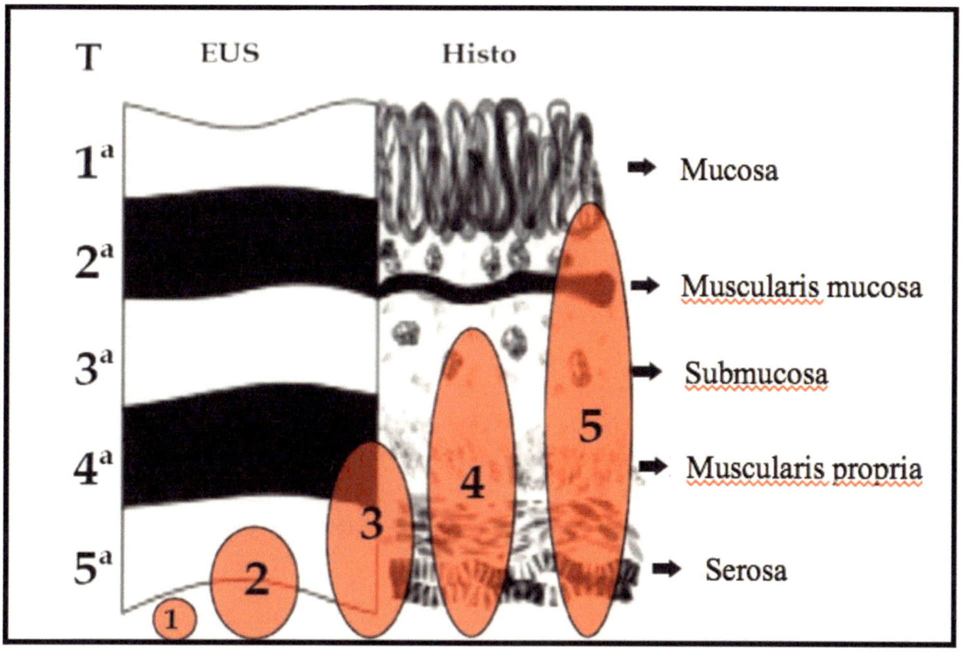

Figure 1. Depth of endometriosis invasion in intestinal wall according to the echo-logic classification. The acronym EUS indicates a schematic representation of the five layers of the intestinal wall, identified during endoscopic ultrasound. The acronym HISTO is a histological correlation of the layers of the wall, evidenced in EUS. "1" = extra-intestinal endometriosis; "2" = endometriosis into the serosa; "3" = endometriosis into the muscularis propria; "4" = endometriosis into the submucosa; and "5" = endometriosis into the mucosa.

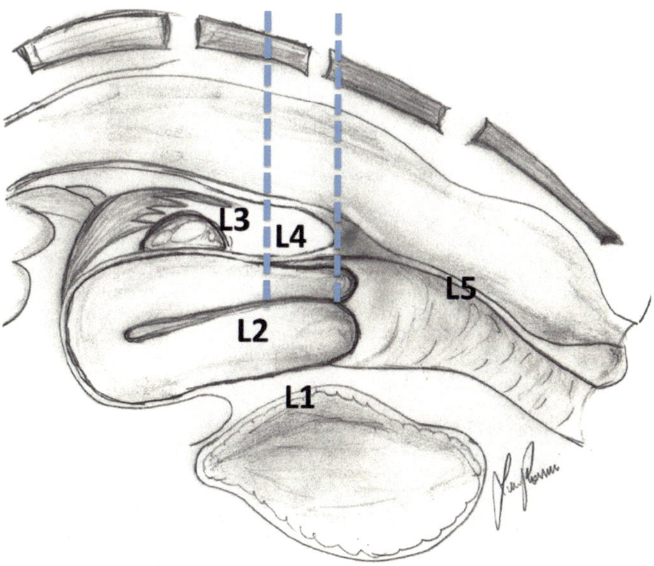

Figure 2. Schematic representation—location of endometriotic nodes in the pelvis according to echo-logic classification. "1" = pre-cervical endometriosis; "2" = paracervical endometriosis (right or left); "3" = node retrocervical endometriosis; "4" = endometriosis of rectovaginal nodules in reflection; and "5" = rectovaginal septum.

"ue," lowercase, precede each penetration stage. Then, the letter "T," uppercase preceding the number, indicates the degree of penetration, or not, of the intestinal wall, and lastly, the letter "L," uppercase, precedes the number to indicate the position of the lesion in the pelvis [3, 6].

Deep lesions tend to have a nodular pattern with a "C" shape (**Figure 3**); however, there are infiltrative lesions that take a pattern of longitudinal growth, and others have a mixed pattern. In peritoneal cavity, intestinal lesions may adhere to other organs and structures leading to the formation of blocks usually involving the uterus and/or the ovaries [3].

1.3. Clinical manifestations

The main clinical gynecologic manifestations include chronic pelvic pain, back pain, menstrual disorders, and infertility. Over 60% of women with endometriosis have chronic intestinal symptoms. Diarrhea, constipation, tenesmus, nausea, vomiting, fever, anorexia, weight loss, and hematochezia may be present at different intensities. Even without parietal invasion, an endometriotic lesion adjacent to any intestinal segment may cause digestive symptoms. Some women may also be asymptomatic [1, 4].

1.4. Clinical evaluation

The complexity of the disease is determined by the variety of clinical presentations: the multifocality, the involvement of non-gynecological sites, and the difficulty in the diagnosis of

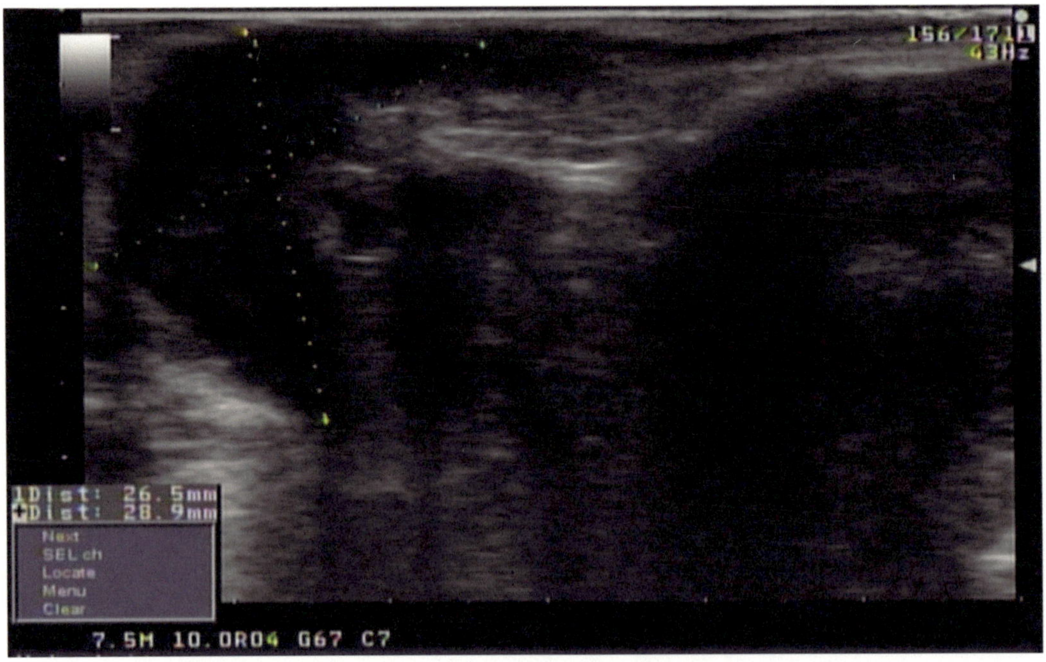

Figure 3. Endometriotic lesion, hypoechogenic and heterogeneous, infiltrating the intestinal wall (ueT4L3).

the disease by preoperative imaging examinations and in the definition of the proper surgical treatment [5].

Clinical evaluation is performed as part of the overall assessment of a patient who presents with pelvic pain and/or infertility.

2. Imaging diagnosis and treatment

Gynecological pelvic exam is considered important for evaluating the extent of pelvic lesions. Through vaginal and rectal touch examination, thickening or nodularity in the pouch of Douglas, uterosacral ligaments, and/or the rectovaginal septum are the most significant data. However, the absence of positive signs does not rule out the disease [1].

Although considered important, gynecological pelvic exam is not sufficient for the diagnosis of the location of deeply infiltrating endometriosis [5]. Imaging methods can suggest the diagnosis of endometriosis and help to map the disease [1, 7].

Some imaging methods can provide answers to these questions:

1. Is there an infiltration compromising the intestinal wall?
2. What is the location of the endometriosis lesion?
3. What is the depth, the extension, and the fraction of the circumference of the intestinal wall invaded?
4. Is there invasion of adjacent organs or structures and adhesions in the cavity?
5. What is the distance between the lesion and the peritoneal reflection?
6. What is the distance between the lesion and the anal sphincter?
7. Is the rectovaginal septum compromised?
8. Is the disease multifocal?
9. Is there another type of intestinal lesion mimicking intestinal endometriosis?
10. Is histologic differential diagnosis necessary?

A study showed that TVUS had better sensitivity, specificity, and accuracy in deep retrocervical and rectosigmoid endometriosis when compared with MRI and gynecological examination [8].

Another study compared diagnostic accuracy of physical examination, transvaginal ultrasound (TVUS), transrectal ultrasound (TRUS), and MRI in the evaluation of deep infiltrating endometriosis. The study concluded that MRI gives similar results to TVUS and TRUS for the diagnosis of intestinal endometriosis but has higher sensitivity and likelihood ratios of uterosacral ligament and vaginal involvement [9]. However, some studies showed that TRUS and TVUS were superior to MRI for detecting lesions in rectosigmoid. The TVUS should be used as the first-line imaging study [10, 11].

MRI is very useful in the complete evaluation of the pelvis (pelvic floor, bladder, ureter, and muscles). It is the best option for the evaluation of ovarian endometriosis, and it has good accuracy in the diagnosis of deep implants of the intestinal wall or rectovaginal septum [1, 12].

Colonoscopy is often performed in many patients with endometriosis, especially in patients with intestinal symptoms such as rectal bleeding. However, only 50% of deep intestinal lesions have specific signs of endometriosis such as subephitelial lesions, which promote deformation and reduction in the lumen (**Figure 4**). Frequently, there is a paucity of mucosal involvement. A prospective study showed colonoscopic findings suggestive of intestinal endometriosis in 4% of cases. Colonoscopy failed to diagnose intestinal endometriosis in 92% of patients who underwent surgery. So, this invasive procedure should not be routinely performed in the diagnosis of intestinal endometriosis [13]. On the other hand, it should be routinely used to exclude other intestinal diseases of the rectum, colon, and terminal ileum that can mimic intestinal symptoms of endometriosis (present in around 60% of patients with deep endometriosis).

When histological confirmation of intestinal endometriosis is necessary, TRUS-FNA is considered a safe procedure. In 2010, Rossini performed TRUS-FNA in 85 patients with suspected endometriotic lesions and characterized the histological findings of endometriosis in 97% of the patients [14]. Puncture was restricted only to lesions that compromise at least the muscular layer of the intestinal wall (ueT3) [3]. The hypothetical risk of seeding endometriotic cells was avoided because TRUS-FNA was performed without the penetration of the peritoneal cavity, and no other organs were transfixed. Histological diagnosis using TVUS-FNA still presents limitations, that is, the risk of peritoneal and/or vaginal implants in the path of the needle.

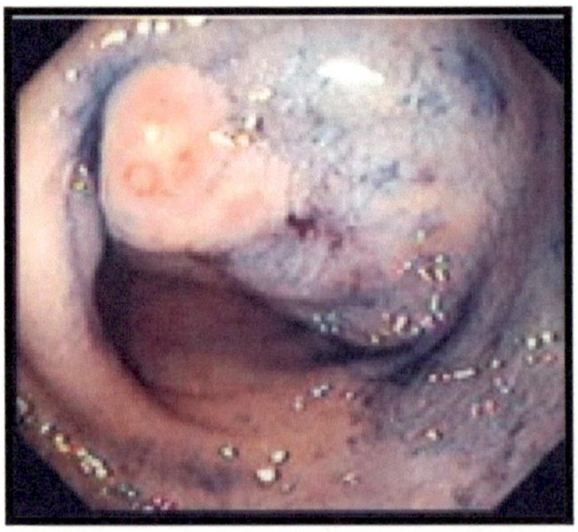

Figure 4. Colonoscopy image—endometriotic lesion infiltrating the intestinal wall.

2.1. Transrectal ultrasound

The TRUS has been used for more than a decade for the diagnosis and staging of deep endometriosis, providing relevant data for surgical treatment. It is useful to determine the depth of infiltration and the distance from the anal junction. Evaluation of intestinal endometriosis can be performed by using rigid linear probes (**Figure 5**), linear probes, or radial echoendoscopes.

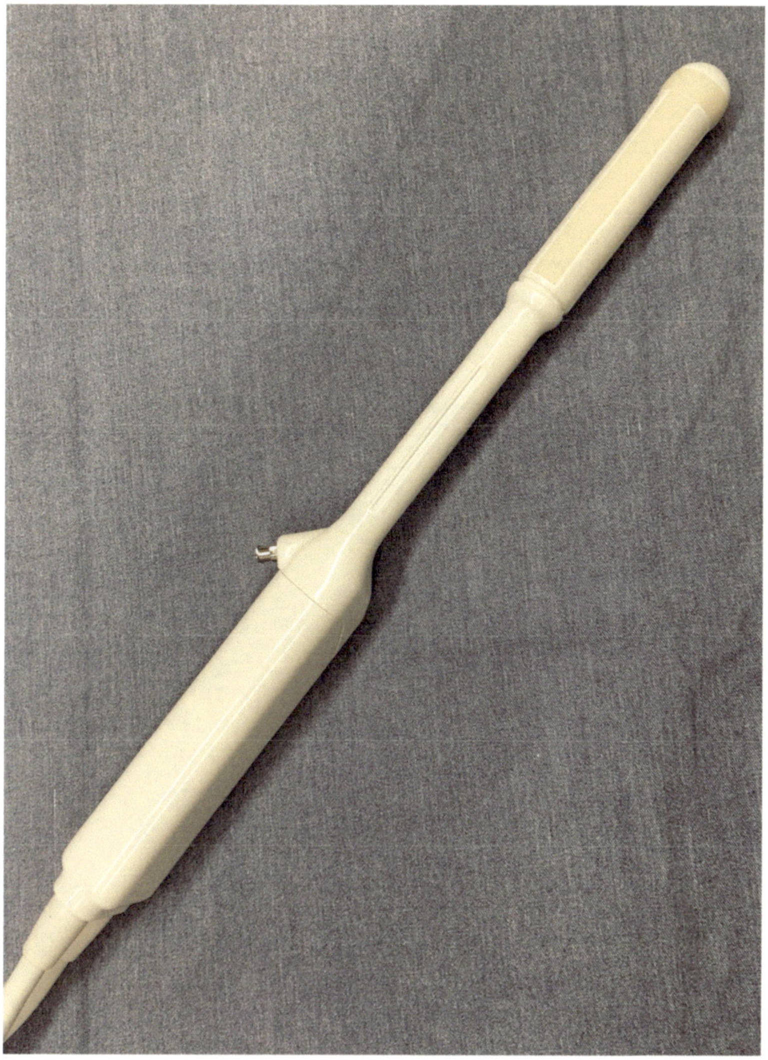

Figure 5. Rigid probe (Hitachi EUP U533).

The rigid probe facilitates the evaluation of lesions located in the rectosigmoid and rectovaginal septum [3]. Using rigid probes, the patient should be positioned in the left lateral decubitus with flexion of the thighs and legs. First, a deep rectal touch examination should be performed to check for anorectal stenosis and/or nodules in the regions of the anus, rectum, rectovaginal septum, pouch of Douglas, cervix, and paracervical regions. Subsequently, the rigid probe should be introduced through the anus and immediately pointed to the back of the patient. The probe should then be softly slid over the sacrum for up to approximately 7–10 cm in the rectal lumen. At this point, a balloon coupled over the probe is filled with water (at least 40 mL). The probe is then pushed up gently with short up and down movements until the distal sigmoid colon. In this position, the right and left iliac vessels and sometimes the bifurcation of abdominal aorta and the right kidney can be observed. Evaluation of the intestinal wall and surrounding tissues, including pelvic organs and iliac vessels, is performed using movements of introduction, traction, and rotation of the probe on its longitudinal axis (clockwise and counterclockwise), as well as by compression or decompression of the transducer against the wall [3].

The presence of hypoechogenic, irregular, homogeneous, or heterogeneous lesions, around or infiltrating pelvic structures, or the intestinal wall are considered suspect of endometriosis (**Figures 6–8**).

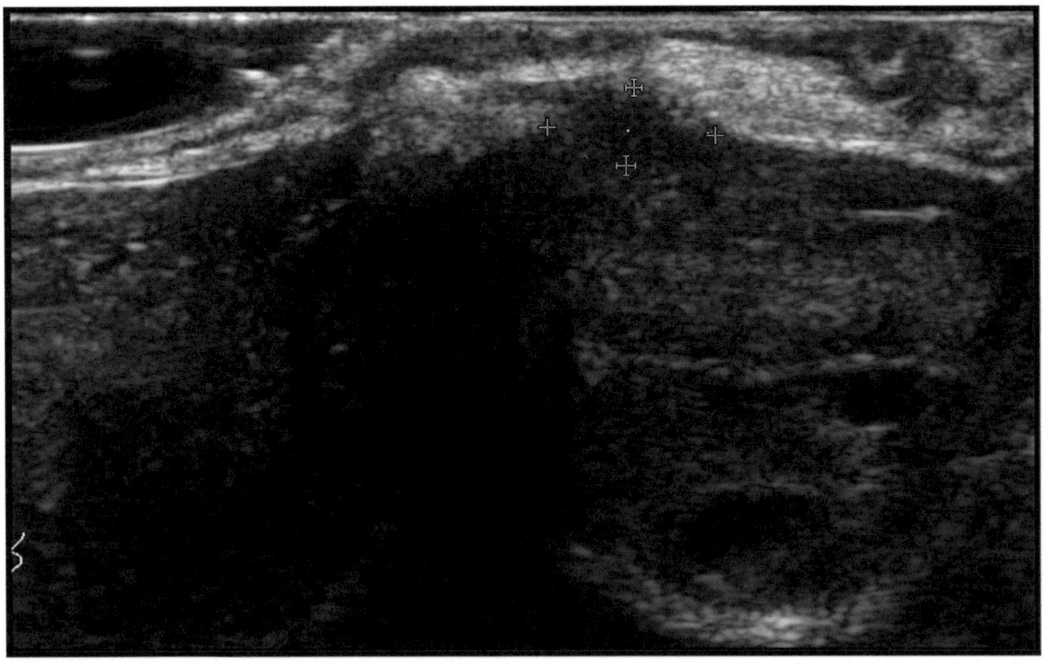

Figure 6. Extra-intestinal endometriotic lesion (ueT1L2 R).

http://dx.doi.org/10.5772/66080

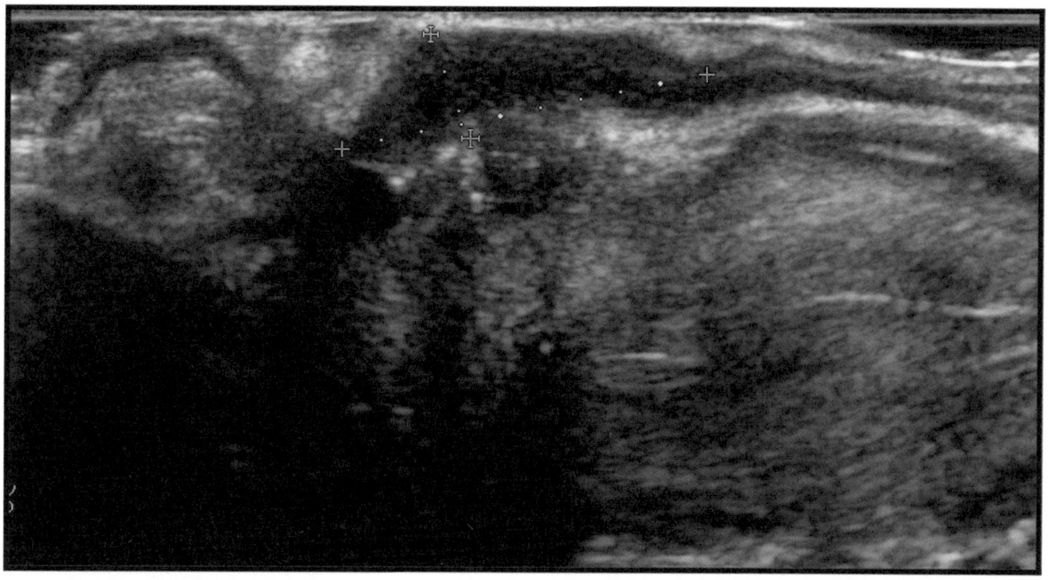

Figure 7. Hypoechogenic and heterogeneous lesion, infiltrating the intestinal wall (ueT3L3).

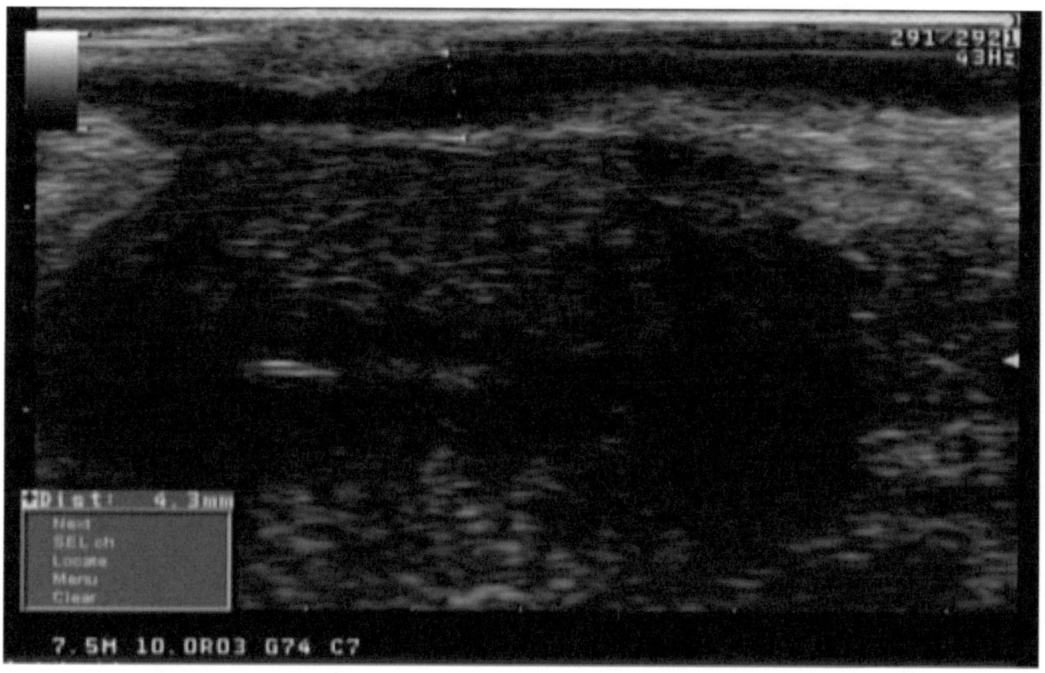

Figure 8. Endometriotic lesion (ueT3L3).

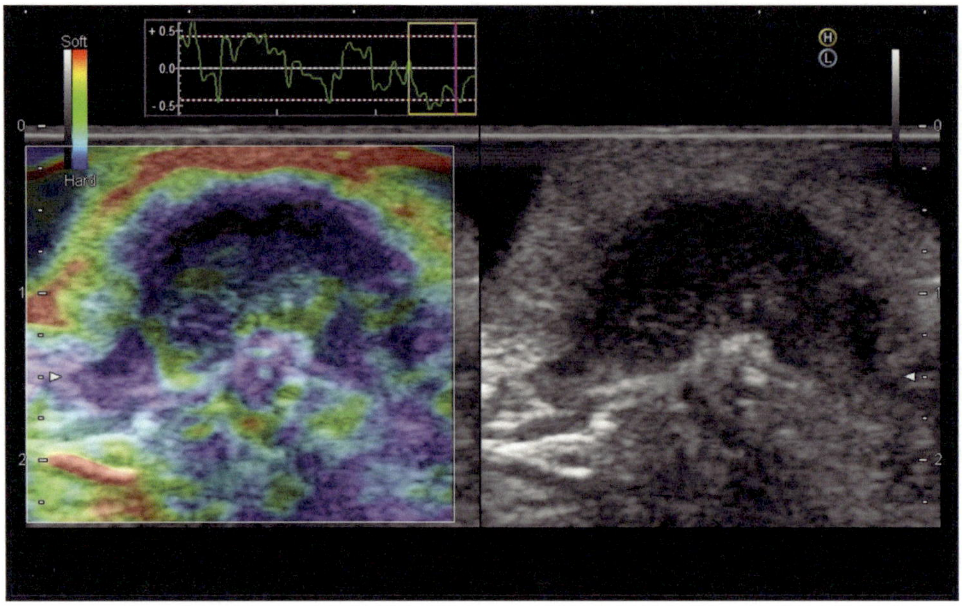

Figure 9. TRUS—Endometriotic lesion (ueT3L4) using transrectal ultrasound and elastography.

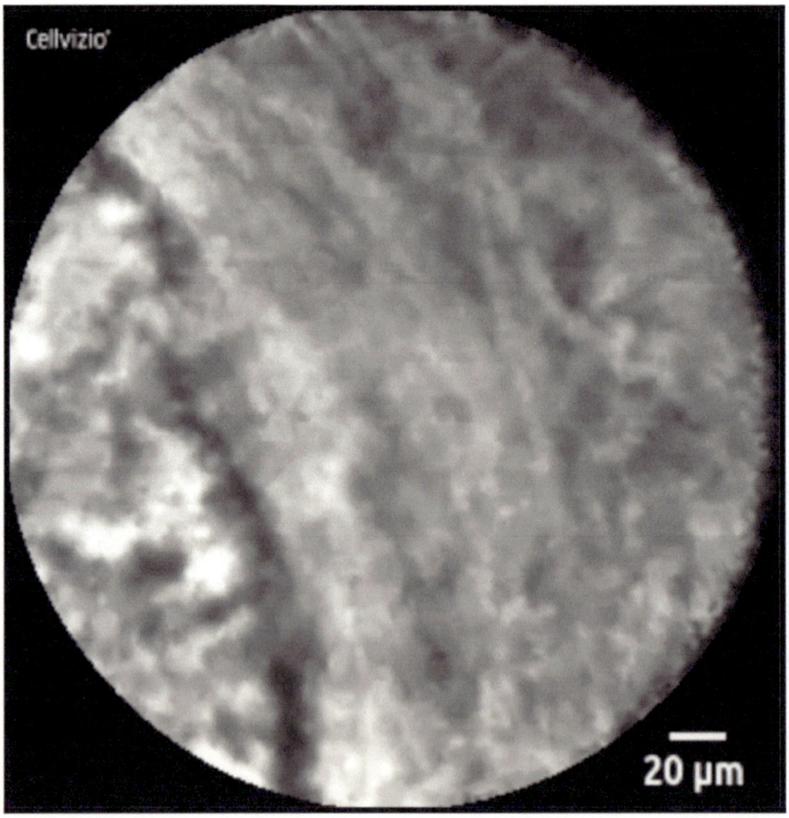

Figure 10. Confocal—endometrial stroma (grayish spots in the middle of fibrosis).

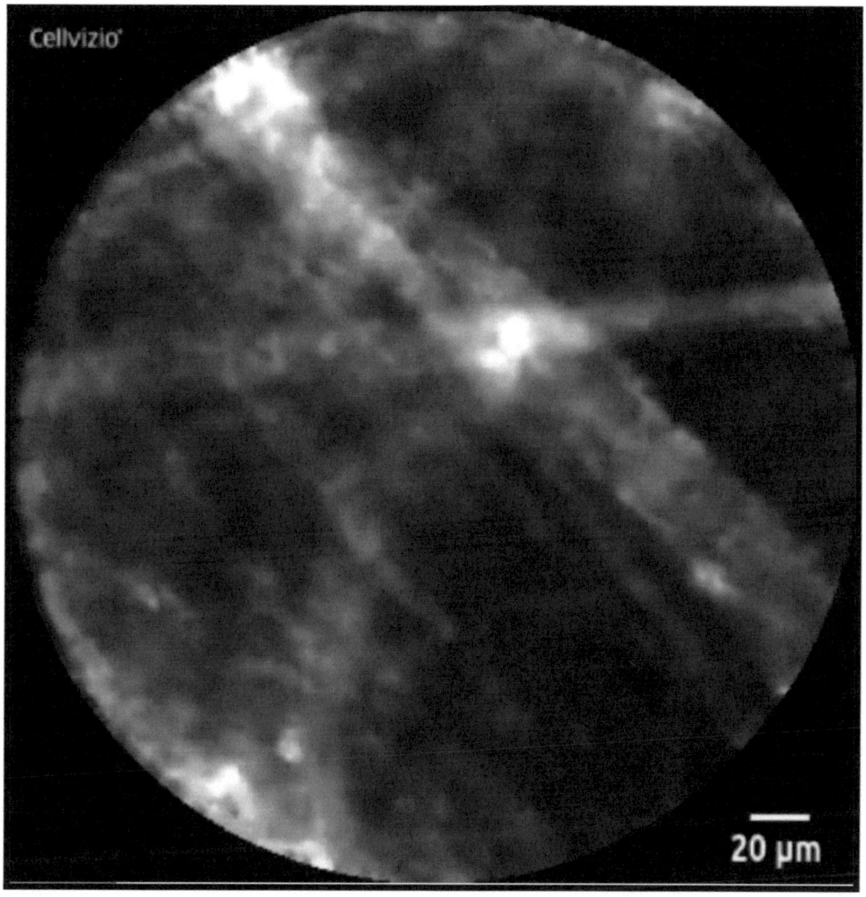

Figure 11. Confocal—fibrous (elongated grayish fibers).

Studies focusing on elastography (**Figure 9**) and confocal laser endomicroscopy (**Figures 10–12**) have been used to improve the accuracy of TRUS for the diagnosis of deep pelvic endometriosis with rectal involvement.

2.2. Treatment

Clinical treatment, exclusive for deep pelvic endometriosis, is still controversial. Medical therapy treats all sites of disease simultaneously, but systemic adverse effects may occur and also recurrence of symptoms when the use of medication is discontinued [4].

Surgical treatment may be the best option in some cases, because it promotes complete excision of the endometriosis lesions [4]. The recent trend is to prefer nodule excision, when feasible, rather than radical digestive resection; therefore, it is important to take into consideration the staging of rectal and sigmoid infiltrating endometriosis in the preoperative clinical evaluation [15]. At the presence of lesions in the intestinal or urinary organs, a gastrointestinal or urologic surgeon is respectively recommended [1].

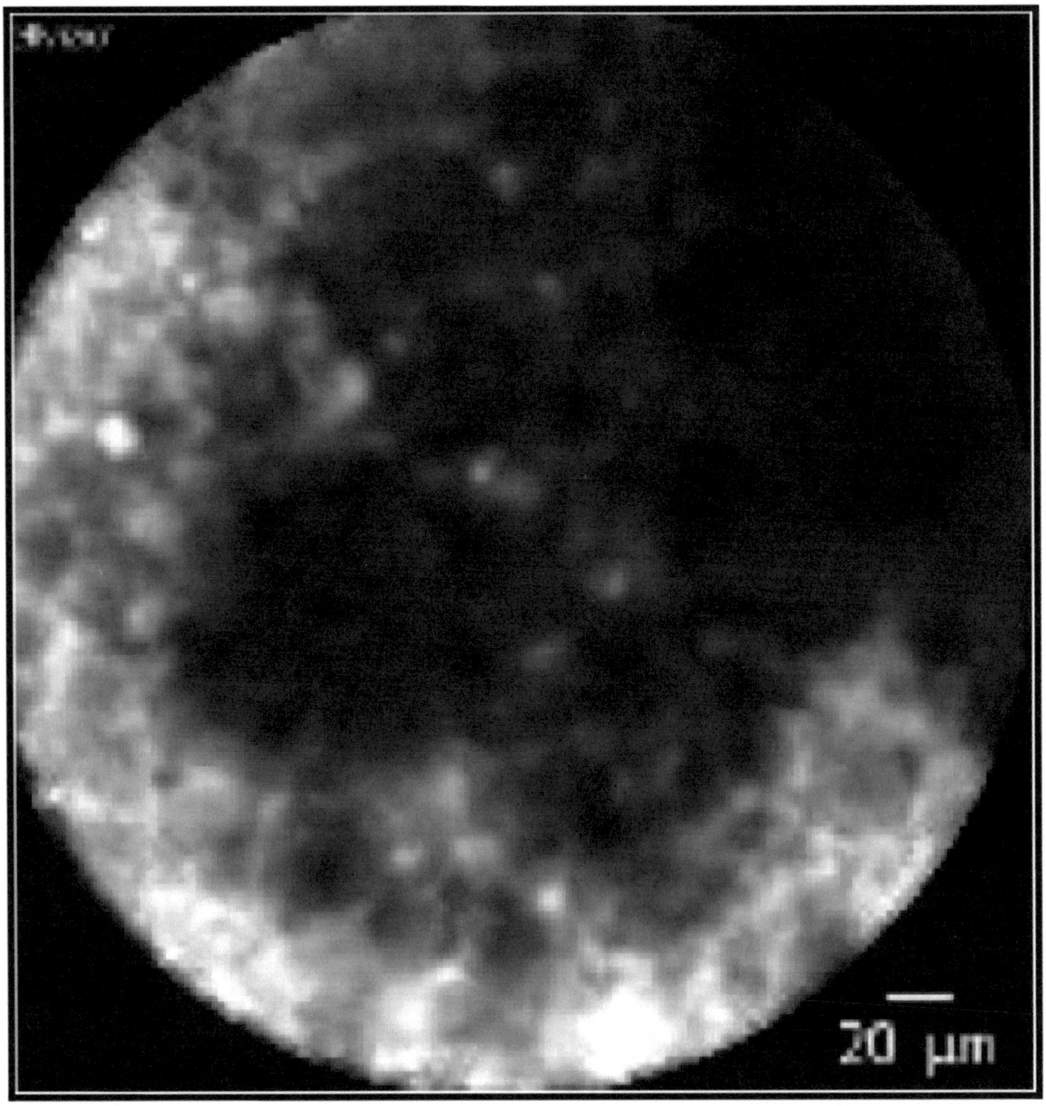

Figure 12. Endometrial glands (dark clouds).

3. Final considerations

Endometriosis is a costly chronic disease causing pelvic pain and infertility and may hence impair quality of life. All women presenting with these symptoms should be evaluated for endometriosis. TRUS is not considered the first-line option to evaluate intestinal endometriosis, but it is essential to determine the depth of infiltration and the distance from the anal junction. This information is useful to assess the extent of rectal surgery [4].

http://dx.doi.org/10.5772/66080

The treatment of deep pelvic endometriosis with intestinal involvement should be individualized and performed by a multidisciplinary team including gynecologists, psychologists, and surgeons with training and experience in advanced techniques of laparoscopic surgery.

Author details

Lucio Giovanni Battista Rossini*, Juliana Marques Drigo and Gisele de Fatima Cordeiro Leite

*Address all correspondence to: luciorossini@uol.com.br

Hospital Sírio-Libanês and Santa Casa de São Paulo, São Paulo (SP), Brazil

References

[1] Rossini LG, Ribeiro PA, Rodrigues FC, Filippi SS, Zago RR, Schneider NC, Okawa L, Klug WA. Transrectal ultrasound—techniques and outcomes in the management of intestinal endometriosis. Endosc Ultrasound. 2012; 1: 23–35. doi:10.7178/eus.01.005

[2] Nisenblat V, Bossuyt PMM, Farquhar C, Johnson N, Hull ML. Imaging modalities for the non-invasive diagnosis of endometriosis. Cochrane Database Syst Rev. 2016; Issue 2: CD009591. doi:10.1002/14651858.CD009591.pub

[3] Rossini LGB. Endometriose intestinal. In: Averbach M, Corrêa P, editors. Colonoscopia. 2nd ed. Rio de Janeiro: Revinter; 2014. pp. 285–292.

[4] Berlanda N, Vercellini P, Fedele L. Endometriosis of bowel or rectovaginal space [Internet]. 2016. Available from: http://www.uptodate.com/contents/endometriosis-of-bowel-or-rectovaginal-space [Accessed: 2016-04-06].

[5] Trippia CH, Zomer MT, Terazaki CR, Martin RL, Ribeiro R, Kondo W. Relevance of Imaging Examinations in the Surgical Planning of Patients with Bowel Endometriosis. Clin Med Insights Reprod Health. 2016; 10: 1–8. doi:10.4137/CMRH. S29472

[6] Ribeiro PAG, Almeida-Prado RA, Aoki T, et al. The echo-logic for deep pelvic endometriosis. J Am Assoc Gynecol Laparosc. 2002; 9(3 Suppl): S74. doi:10.1016/S1074-3804(02)80243-2

[7] Philip CA, Bisch C, Coulon A, de Saint-Hilaire P, Rudigoz RC, Dubernard G. Correlation between three-dimensional rectosonography and magnetic resonance imaging in the diagnosis of rectosigmoid endometriosis: a preliminary study on the first fifty cases. Eur J Obstet Gynecol Reprod Biol. 2015; 187: 35–40. doi:10.1016/j.ejogrb.2015.02.006

[8] Abrao MS, Gonçalves MO, Dias JA Jr, Podgaec S, Chamie LP, Blasbalg R. Comparison between clinical examination, transvaginal sonography and magnetic resonance imaging for the diagnosis of deep endometriosis. Hum Reprod. 2007; 22: 3092–3097

[9] Bazot M, Lafont C, Rouzier R, Roseau G, Thomassin-Naggara I, Daraï E. Diagnostic accuracy of physical examination, transvaginal sonography, rectal endoscopic sonography, and magnetic resonance imaging to diagnose deep infiltrating endometriosis. Fertil Steril. 2009; 92: 1825–1833. doi:10.1016/j.fertnstert.2008.09.00

[10] Bazot M, Detchev R, Cortez A, Amouyal P, Uzan S, Daraï E. Transvaginal sonography and rectal endoscopic sonography for the assessment of pelvic endometriosis: a preliminary comparison. Hum Reprod. 2003; 18: 1686–1692. doi:10.1093/humrep/deg314

[11] Bazot M, Malzy P, Cortez A, Roseau G, Amouyal P, Daraï E. Accuracy of transvaginal sonography and rectal endoscopic sonography in the diagnosis of deep infiltrating endometriosis. Ultrasound Obstet Gynecol. 2007; 30: 994–1001. doi:10.1002/uog.4070

[12] Chapron C, Vieira M, Chopin N, et al. Accuracy of rectal endoscopic ultrasonography and magnetic resonance imaging in the diagnosis of rectal involvement for patients presenting with deeply infiltrating endometriosis. Ultrasound Obstet Gynecol 2004; 24: 175–1759.

[13] Milone M, Mollo A1, Musella M, Maietta P, Sosa Fernandez LM, Shatalova O, Conforti A, Barone G, De Placido G, Milone F. Role of colonoscopy in the diagnostic work-up of bowel endomet'riosis. World J Gastroenterol. 2015; 21: 4997–5001. doi:10.3748/wjg.v21.i16.4997

[14] Rossini LGB. Sensibility and technical application of fine needle aspiration (FNA) guided by intestinal endosonography for histological diagnosis of deep endometriosis located in rectum and distal sigmoid [thesis]. Faculdade de Ciências Médicas da Santa Casa de São Paulo; 2010.

[15] Roseau G. Recto-sigmoid endoscopic-ultrasonography in the staging of deep infiltrating endometriosis. World J Gastrointest Endosc. 2014; 6: 525–533. doi:10.4253/wjge.v6.i11.525